T0362400

Advances in Systemic Therapy for Non-Small Cell Lung Cancer

Editors

JESSICA S. DONINGTON
JYOTI D. PATEL

THORACIC SURGERY CLINICS

www.thoracic.theclinics.com

Consulting Editor
M. BLAIR MARSHALL

May 2020 • Volume 30 • Number 2

ELSEVIER

1600 John F. Kennedy Boulevard • Suite 1800 • Philadelphia, Pennsylvania, 19103-2899

http://www.thoracic.theclinics.com

THORACIC SURGERY CLINICS Volume 30, Number 2
May 2020 ISSN 1547-4127, ISBN-13: 978-0-323-79189-2

Editor: John Vassallo (j.vassallo@elsevier.com)
Developmental Editor: Laura Fisher

Thoracic Surgery Clinics (ISSN 1547-4127) is published quarterly by Elsevier Inc., 360 Park Avenue South, New York, NY 10010-1710. Months of publication are February, May, August, and November. Business and editorial offices: 1600 John F. Kennedy Boulevard, Suite 1800, Philadelphia, PA 19103-2899. Periodicals postage paid at New York, NY, and additional mailing offices. Subscription prices are $393.00 per year (US individuals), $623.00 per year (US institutions), $100.00 per year (US students), $460.00 per year (Canadian individuals), $806.00 per year (Canadian institutions), $100.00 per year (Canadian students), $225.00 per year (international students), $480.00 per year (international individuals), and $806.00 per year (international institutions). Foreign air speed delivery is included in all Clinics' subscription prices. All prices are subject to change without notice. **POSTMASTER:** Send address changes to Thoracic Surgery Clinics, Elsevier Health Sciences Division, Subscription Customer Service, 3251 Riverport Lane, Maryland Heights, MO 63043. **Customer Service (orders, claims, online, change of address): Telephone: 1-800-654-2452 (U.S. and Canada); 314-447-8871 (outside U.S. and Canada). Fax: 314-447-8029. E-mail: journalscustomerservice-usa@elsevier.com (for print support); journalsonlinesupport-usa@elsevier.com (for online support).**

Reprints. For copies of 100 or more, of articles in this publication, please contact Commercial Rights Department, Elsevier Inc., 360 Park Avenue South, New York, NY 10010-1710. Tel: 212-633-3874; Fax: 212-633-3820; E-mail: reprints@elsevier.com.

Thoracic Surgery Clinics is covered in *MEDLINE/PubMed (Index Medicus), EMBASE/Excerpta Medica, Science Citation Index Expanded (SciSearch®), Journal Citation Reports/Science Edition,* and *Current Contents®/Clinical Medicine*.

Contributors

CONSULTING EDITOR

M. BLAIR MARSHALL, MD, FACS
Associate Chief for Quality and Safety, Division of Thoracic Surgery, Brigham and Women's Hospital, Associate Professor of Surgery, Harvard Medical School, Boston, Massachusetts

EDITORS

JESSICA S. DONINGTON, MD, MSCR
Professor of Surgery, Chief, Section of General Thoracic Surgery, University of Chicago, Chicago, Illinois

JYOTI D. PATEL, MD
Professor of Medicine, Associate Vice Chair for Clinical Research, Department of Medicine, Northwestern University, Chicago, Illinois

AUTHORS

LYUDMILA BAZHENOVA, MD
Professor of Medicine, Division of Hematology and Oncology, Department of Medicine, University of California, San Diego, La Jolla, California

CHRISTINE M. BESTVINA, MD
Assistant Professor, Department of Medicine, Section of Hematology/Oncology, University of Chicago Medicine, Chicago, Illinois

HOSSEIN BORGHAEI, DO, MS
Chief, Division of Thoracic Medical Oncology, Professor, Department of Hematology/Oncology, Fox Chase Cancer Center, Philadelphia, Pennsylvania

STEPHEN R. BRODERICK, MD, MPHS, FACS
Assistant Professor, Department of Surgery, Johns Hopkins Medical Institutions, Baltimore, Maryland

JEAN G. BUSTAMANTE-ALVAREZ, MD, MS
Chief Hematology/Oncology Fellow, Division of Medical Oncology, Department of Internal Medicine, Ohio State University Wexner Medical Center, Columbus, Ohio

AMANDA S. CASS, PharmD, BCPS, BCOP
Clinical Pharmacist Specialist, Thoracic Oncology, Department of Pharmaceutical Sciences, Vanderbilt Ingram Cancer Center, Vanderbilt University Medical Center, Nashville, Tennessee

AADEL A. CHAUDHURI, MD, PhD
Assistant Professor, Department of Radiation Oncology, Washington University School of Medicine, St Louis, Missouri

RE-I. CHIN, MD
Resident Physician, Department of Radiation Oncology, Washington University School of Medicine, St Louis, Missouri

KELLY FITZGERALD, MD, PhD
Resident Physician, Department of Radiation Oncology, Memorial Sloan Kettering Cancer Center, New York, New York

RYAN D. GENTZLER, MD, MS
Assistant Professor, UVA Cancer Center, Division of Hematology/Oncology, University

of Virginia School of Medicine, Charlottesville, Virginia

NICHOLAS P. GIUSTINI, MD
Hematology and Oncology Fellow, Division of Hematology and Oncology, Department of Medicine, University of California, San Diego, La Jolla, California

JESSICA A. HELLYER, MD
Department of Medicine, Division of Oncology, Stanford Cancer Institute, Stanford University School of Medicine, Stanford, California

LEORA HORN, MD, MSc, FRCPC
Associate Professor of Medicine, Ingram Associate Professor of Cancer Research, Vanderbilt Ingram Cancer Center, Vanderbilt University Medical Center, Nashville, Tennessee

MELINDA L. HSU, MD
Department of Oncology, Sidney Kimmel Comprehensive Cancer Center, Bloomberg-Kimmel Institute for Cancer Immunotherapy, Johns Hopkins University, Baltimore, Maryland

PAUL A. JONES, BS
Graduate Student, Department of Radiation Oncology, Division of Molecular Cell Biology, Washington University School of Medicine, St Louis, Missouri

JULIA JUDD, DO
Fellow, Department of Hematology/Oncology, Fox Chase Cancer Center, Philadelphia, Pennsylvania

ERIN M. McLOUGHLIN, MD
Clinical Fellow, Division of Hematology/ Oncology, University of Virginia School of Medicine, Charlottesville, Virginia

JARUSHKA NAIDOO, MBBCH, MHS
Department of Oncology, Sidney Kimmel Comprehensive Cancer Center, Bloomberg-Kimmel Institute for Cancer Immunotherapy, Johns Hopkins University, Baltimore, Maryland

DWIGHT H. OWEN, MD, MS
Assistant Professor of Internal Medicine, Division of Medical Oncology, Department of Internal Medicine, Ohio State University Wexner Medical Center, Columbus, Ohio

BRUNA PELLINI, MD
Clinical Fellow, Department of Medicine, Division of Oncology, Washington University School of Medicine, St Louis, Missouri

KAREN L. RECKAMP, MD, MS
Cedars-Sinai Medical Center, Los Angeles, California

ANTHONY V. SERRITELLA, MD
Department of Medicine, University of Chicago Medicine, Chicago, Illinois

CHARLES B. SIMONE II, MD
Professor and Full Member, Department of Radiation Oncology, Memorial Sloan Kettering Cancer Center, New York Proton Center, New York, New York

JEFFREY SZYMANSKI, MD, PhD
Bioinformatics Scientist, Department of Radiation Oncology, Washington University School of Medicine, St Louis, Missouri

HEATHER A. WAKELEE, MD
Department of Medicine, Division of Oncology, Stanford Cancer Institute, Stanford University School of Medicine, Stanford, California

Contents

Erratum xi

Preface: The Rapidly Changing World of Thoracic Oncology xiii

Jessica S. Donington and Jyoti D. Patel

Current Landscape of Personalized Therapy 121

Leora Horn and Amanda S. Cass

Almost a half of patients diagnosed with non-small cell lung cancer (NSCLC) present with incurable disease, and a significant number of patients who are treated with curative intent for early-stage disease will eventually recur. Systemic therapy is selected based on tumor histology, squamous versus nonsquamous NSCLC, molecular testing, and PD-L1 score. Depending on PD-L1 score, patients are eligible for immunotherapy alone or in combination with chemotherapy in the first-line setting. Oncogenic driver mutations can be detected in approximately 50% of patients with nonsquamous NSCLC of which several can be targeted therapeutically with small molecular inhibitors. Continued research is needed for more specific agents with less toxicity and better central nervous system penetration, and agents to treat patients who develop resistance against targeted treatments and immunotherapy.

Epidermal Growth Factor Receptor Mutations 127

Erin M. McLoughlin and Ryan D. Gentzler

Up to 20% of lung adenocarcinomas in the United States and Europe and 50% in Asia have activating mutations of the tyrosine kinase domain of the epidermal growth factor receptor (EGFR). The identification and subsequent targeting of mutations with EGFR–tyrosine kinase inhibitors (TKIs) led to significant advances in treatment of EGFR-mutant lung cancer. Newer-generation EGFR-TKIs resulted in improvement in outcomes, with less toxic side effects and better tolerability. Resistance to EGFR-TKIs remains a significant barrier, and better understanding of resistance mechanisms is needed. Efforts are ongoing to incorporate targeted therapy into treatment of patients with earlier-stage disease.

Anaplastic Lymphoma Kinase Mutation–Positive Non–Small Cell Lung Cancer 137

Anthony V. Serritella and Christine M. Bestvina

The treatment of patients with advanced non–small cell lung cancer with anaplastic lymphoma kinase chromosomal rearrangements has been revolutionized by the development of tyrosine kinase inhibitors (TKIs). Excellent progress has been made over the past decade, with 4 TKIs now approved in the front-line setting. Alectinib is the preferred first-line option based on its efficacy and side-effect profile. The central nervous system (CNS) activity of alectinib and brigatinib has allowed for treatment of CNS metastases with TKI therapy. Once resistance inevitably develops, newer therapies such as lorlatinib can be considered.

ROS1-rearranged Non–Small Cell Lung Cancer 147

Nicholas P. Giustini and Lyudmila Bazhenova

ROS1-rearranged non–small cell lung cancer (NSCLC) makes up approximately 1% to 2% of all NSCLC, is oncogenically driven by a constitutively activated ROS1 kinase paired with certain fusion partners, and can be detected by several different assays. These patients are initially treated with tyrosine kinase inhibitors (TKIs), which target the activated ROS1 kinase. Eventually these tumors develop resistance to initial TKI treatment through secondary kinase mutations that block TKI binding or activation of bypass signaling pathways, which subvert ROS1 as the driver of the malignancy. Investigation of several TKIs that have shown efficacy in secondary resistant patients is underway.

Molecular Targets Beyond the Big 3 157

Karen L. Reckamp

Lung cancer is a heterogeneous genomic disease. Smoking remains the primary cause. Genetic susceptibility and environmental exposures are responsible for 10% to 15% of cases. Targeted therapies improve survival in patients with tumors with oncogenic drivers. It is critical to expand our understanding of genetic alterations in non-small cell lung cancer to increase the available targeted therapies. Alterations beyond *epidermal growth factor receptor (EGFR), ALK, and ROS1* exemplify lung cancer's complexity and the need for investments in precision therapy to extend patient survival and improve outcomes. This article covers genetic targets beyond *EGFR, ALK and ROS1*, their novel agents, challenges, and future directions.

Liquid Biopsies Using Circulating Tumor DNA in Non-Small Cell Lung Cancer 165

Bruna Pellini, Jeffrey Szymanski, Re-I. Chin, Paul A. Jones, and Aadel A. Chaudhuri

Liquid biopsies for the diagnosis and treatment of lung cancer have developed rapidly, driven primarily by technical advances in sensitivity to detect circulating tumor DNA (ctDNA). Still, technical limitations such as the challenge of detecting low-level ctDNA variants and distinguishing tumor-related variants from clonal hematopoiesis remain. With further technical advancements, new applications for ctDNA analysis are emerging including detection of post-treatment molecular residual disease (MRD), clinical trial selection, and early cancer detection. This chapter reviews the current state of ctDNA testing in NSCLC, the underlying technological advances enabling ctDNA detection, and the potential to expand ctDNA analysis to new applications.

Adjuvant Chemotherapy 179

Jessica A. Hellyer and Heather A. Wakelee

Five-year survival rates for patients with early-stage non–small cell lung cancer have room for improvement. Adjuvant chemotherapy results in a small but significant increase in overall survival at 5 years. Efforts to improve outcomes by intensifying adjuvant treatment, utilizing cancer-specific vaccines or tyrosine kinase inhibitors in unselected patients, have been unsuccessful. In addition to research with immune checkpoint inhibitors that are addressed in a separate article, ongoing studies to personalize adjuvant therapy either by selecting only patients with evidence of minimal residual disease or targeting tumor driver mutations are promising.

Principles of Immunotherapy in Non-Small Cell Lung Cancer 187

Melinda L. Hsu and Jarushka Naidoo

Immunotherapy has transformed the treatment of many tumors. Robust data demonstrating improved overall survival and progression-free survival in patients treated with monoclonal antibodies have established immune checkpoint inhibitors as standard of care in stages III and IV non-small cell lung cancer. Nivolumab is effective in previously treated patients with metastatic non-small cell lung cancer. Pembrolizumab and atezolizumab are approved as monotherapy and in combination with other therapies. Ongoing trials investigate the potential role of immunotherapy in earlier disease settings. Identifying predictive biomarkers of response will further amplify the impact of immune checkpoint inhibitors in the treatment of non-small cell lung cancer.

Combining Immunotherapy and Chemotherapy for Non–Small Cell Lung Cancer 199

Julia Judd and Hossein Borghaei

Over the past year, the combination of platinum-based chemotherapy and immunotherapy has become the standard of care for patients with metastatic non-small cell lung cancer with any programmed death ligand 1 tumor proportion score. There is preclinical evidence demonstrating potential synergistic immunomodulation with combination therapy by enhancing immune-mediated tumor death and by disrupting the immunosuppressive tumor microenvironment that prevents immune detection. This potential synergy or complementary activity has been demonstrated in clinical trials showing improved and durable responses with chemo-immunotherapy.

Biomarkers for Immunotherapy 207

Jean G. Bustamante-Alvarez and Dwight H. Owen

Immune checkpoint inhibitor (ICI) therapy has been approved for several solid tumors, including non–small cell lung cancer. ICIs have shown unprecedented durable responses and higher response rates than chemotherapy in selected patients. The development of biomarkers that serve as predictors of response is crucial for treatment selection. Evidence suggests that the response to immunotherapy depends on tumor genomics and the interactions with the immune system and the tumor microenvironment. This article reviews the data supporting the use of these biomarkers to optimize patient selection for these therapies and explores biomarkers that are the focus of ongoing research.

Adjuvant and Neoadjuvant Immunotherapy in Non–small Cell Lung Cancer 215

Stephen R. Broderick

The advent of immune checkpoint blockade has revolutionized the management of advanced non–small cell lung cancer (NSCLC). Impressive results in the metastatic setting have prompted substantial interest in the application of these agents in earlier-stage disease. Applications of checkpoint blockade in the adjuvant setting are under investigation in several clinical trials. Early trials have demonstrated the safety and feasibility of the administration of checkpoint inhibitors in the neoadjuvant setting. Resection specimens demonstrate encouraging rates of pathologic response. There are several ongoing phase 3 studies comparing neoadjuvant combination chemotherapy and checkpoint blockade to chemotherapy alone in patients with resectable NSCLC.

Combining Immunotherapy with Radiation Therapy in Non–Small Cell Lung Cancer **221**

Kelly Fitzgerald and Charles B. Simone II

Immune checkpoint inhibitors have recently been demonstrated to improve survival in metastatic and locally advanced non-small cell lung cancer (NSCLC). Radiation therapy has a well-established role in the treatment of NSCLC and has more recently been shown to be immunostimulatory, with the potential to enhance the efficacy of immunotherapy. This comprehensive review details the current roles of radiation therapy and immune checkpoint inhibitors in NSCLC, discusses the intersection of these two modalities and their potential to have combined synergistic responses, and highlights existing preclinical and clinical data and ongoing clinical trials of combined immunotherapy and radiotherapy across all NSCLC stages.

THORACIC SURGERY CLINICS

FORTHCOMING ISSUES

August 2020
Peri-operative Management of the Thoracic Patient
Virginia R. Litle and Robert J. Canelli, *Editors*

November 2020
Malignant Pleural Mesothelioma
Bryan M. Burt, *Editor*

February 2021
Thoracic Outlet Syndrome
Dean M. Donahue and Hugh G. Auchincloss, *Editors*

RECENT ISSUES

February 2020
Nonintubated Thoracic Surgery
Vincenzo Ambrogi and Tommaso Claudio Mineo, *Editors*

November 2019
Surgical Management of Paraesophageal Hernia
Inderpal S. Sarkaria and Abbas E. Abbas, *Editors*

August 2019
Thoracic Surgical Education: Current and Future Strategies
Edward D. Verrier, *Editor*

SERIES OF RELATED INTEREST

Surgical Clinics
http://www.surgical.theclinics.com

Surgical Oncology Clinics
http://www.surgonc.theclinics.com

Advances in Surgery
http://www.advancessurgery.com

THE CLINICS ARE AVAILABLE ONLINE!
Access your subscription at:
www.theclinics.com

Erratum

In the article "Results of the National Lung Cancer Screening Trial: Where Are We Now" by Neel P. Chudgar, Peter R. Bucciarelli, Elizabeth M. Jeffries, Nabil P. Rizk, Bernard J. Park, Prasad S. Adusumilli, and David R. Jones, published in the May 2015 issue (Volume 25, Number 2, pages 145–153), under the "Results" section on page 147, the following sentence is incorrect: "False-positive rates were 96.4% in the LDCT group and 95.4% in the CXR group."

The corrected sentence should read: "False discovery rates were 96.4% in the LDCT group and 95.4% in the CXR group."

Thorac Surg Clin 30 (2020) xi
https://doi.org/10.1016/j.thorsurg.2020.02.002

Preface
The Rapidly Changing World of Thoracic Oncology

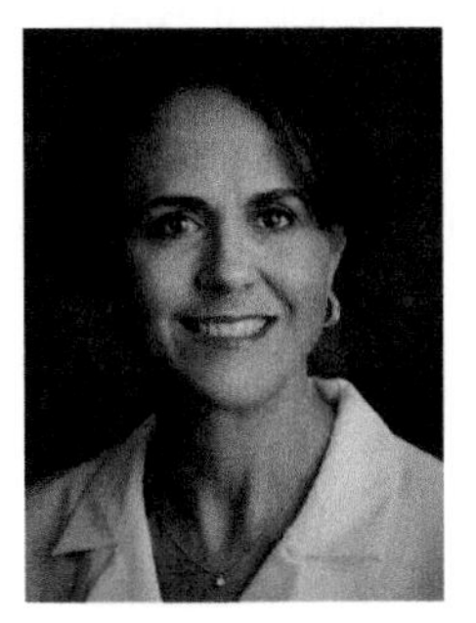

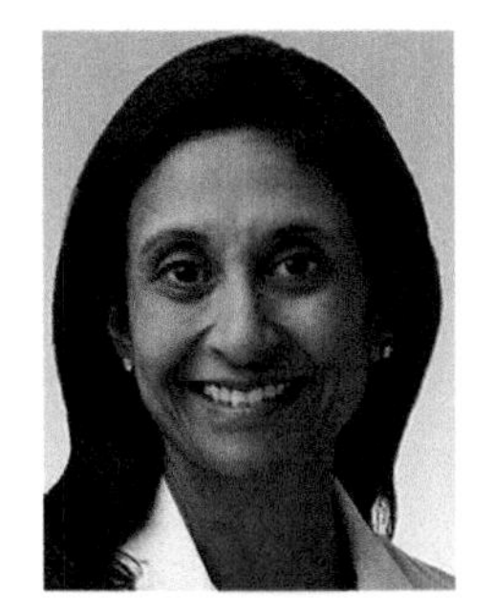

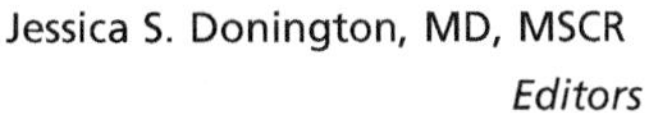

Jessica S. Donington, MD, MSCR   Jyoti D. Patel, MD
Editors

The landscape of care in advanced stage non–small cell lung cancer (NSCLC) is changing at lightning speed. Rarely in oncology have we seen the kind of rapid advancements and broad sweeping changes that are occurring currently in lung cancer. No patient with stage IV NSCLC in 2020 is approached the same way that they would have been 5 years ago. There are entirely new classes of medications, multiple new molecular targets, greater understanding of resistances mechanisms, novel biomarkers, and better tools to track disease response and progression. Subsequently, stage IV NSCLC patients surviving longer than ever and greater numbers presenting to surgeons for consideration of resection as part of these new treatment paradigms. It is important for surgeons to stay abreast of these rapid advances, but it is challenging.

Major changes have occurred in oncogene-addicted NSCLC. Next-generation tyrosine kinase inhibitors have overtaken more established agents as the standard of care in epidermal growth factor receptor (EGFR) and anaplastic lymphoma kinase (ALK)-positive tumors. Multiple mechanisms of acquired resistance have been reported among patients treated with next-generation EGFR tyrosine kinase inhibitors, reflecting the diversity of the landscape with targeted mutations. In addition, new oncogenes, such as mutant BRAF, kinase met gene, and erb-b2 receptor tyrosine kinase 2 gene, and ret protooncogene rearrangements have joined the list of potential targetable drivers. An additional major step forward was the approval of personalized treatment in very uncommon genomic alterations, mainly gene fusions. This raises a new question about the challenge of implementation of next-generation sequencing in daily clinical practice to detect new and uncommon genomic alterations and to capture the heterogeneity of the mechanisms of acquired resistance during treatment.

Immune checkpoint inhibitors (ICIs) are game changers in advanced NSCLC treatment. They are now part of a frontline treatment strategy for almost all patients regardless of histologic subtype. Their use now extends to include stage III disease, shifting prognosis of these patients. Early trials with ICIs as part of induction strategies prior to resection are encouraging, with increased pathologic response rates compared with chemotherapy and no evidence for surgical delay or increase in perioperative complications. Characterization of predictive biomarkers, improved patient selection, definition of strategies upon progression, and prospective evaluation in select subpopulations (such as patients with poor performance status or brain metastases) are on-going challenges.

The field of thoracic oncology has experienced many recent breakthroughs with many promising new therapeutic options. While the breakthroughs have made their initial impact in advanced disease, many are now being investigated in surgically resectable populations. These articles are

Thorac Surg Clin 30 (2020) xiii–xiv
https://doi.org/10.1016/j.thorsurg.2020.02.001
1547-4127/20/© 2020 Published by Elsevier Inc.

thoracic.theclinics.com

designed as a primer to assist thoracic surgical oncologists to stay abreast of these rapid changes in systemic care for NSCLC.

Jessica S. Donington, MD, MSCR
Section of General Thoracic Surgery
University of Chicago
5841 South Maryland Avenue
Room S-546, MC 5047
Chicago, IL 60637, USA

Jyoti D. Patel, MD
Division of Hematology/Oncology
Department of Medicine
Northwestern University
676 North St. Clair Street
Suite 850
Chicago, IL 60611, USA

E-mail addresses:
jdonington@uchicago.edu (J.S. Donington)
jd-patel@northwestern.edu (J.D. Patel)

Current Landscape of Personalized Therapy

Leora Horn, MD, MSc, FRCPC[a], Amanda S. Cass, PharmD, BCPS, BCOP[b,*]

KEYWORDS

- Non–small-cell lung cancer • Immune checkpoint inhibition • Targeted therapies
- Epidermal growth factor receptor • Anaplastic lymphoma kinase

KEY POINTS

- The movement toward personalized medicine has revolutionized treatment strategies for patients with non–small-cell lung cancer.
- Most patients with advanced-stage disease are treated with either targeted therapy or immunotherapy, with chemotherapy alone being used in only select cohorts.
- Immune checkpoint inhibitors are approved by the Food and Drug Administration as first-line and second-line therapy for patients with advanced non–small-cell lung cancer that do not harbor a targetable mutation.
- Patients with a tumor that harbors a mutation should receive targeted therapy directed to their mutation rather than cytotoxic chemotherapy or immunotherapy because targeted therapies are associated with significant tumor regression and decreased toxicity compared with traditional cytotoxic therapy.

INTRODUCTION

Almost a half of the patients diagnosed with non–small-cell lung cancer (NSCLC) present with incurable disease, and a significant number of patients treated with curative intent for early-stage disease will eventually recur. Systemic therapy is given to palliate symptoms, improve quality of life, and prolong survival in patients with advanced-stage disease. Systemic therapy is selected based on tumor histology (squamous vs nonsquamous), results of molecular testing, and programmed cell death ligand 1 (PD-L1) score. The movement toward personalized medicine has revolutionized treatment strategies for patients with NSCLC. Although chemotherapy alone may be appropriate for a very select cohort of patients, most patients with advanced-stage disease will be treated with either targeted therapy or immunotherapy with or without chemotherapy.

All patients with nonsquamous NSCLC and younger patients or never smokers with squamous cell NSCLC should have molecular testing performed on their tumor as part of a comprehensive, large panel. Oncogenic driver mutations can be detected in approximately 50% of patients with nonsquamous NSCLC, several of which can be targeted therapeutically with small molecular inhibitors, including mutations in epidermal growth factor receptor (EGFR) (10%–15%), BRAF (2%), and MET (2%), as well as anaplastic lymphoma kinase (ALK) (5%–7%), ROS1 (1%–2%), NTRK (1%), and RET (1%–2%) fusions. Mutations in KRAS are present in approximately 20% to 25% of patients with NSCLC, and for the first time in clinic we are

[a] Vanderbilt Ingram Cancer Center, Vanderbilt University Medical Center, 2220 Pierce Avenue, 777 Preston Research Building, Nashville, TN 37205, USA; [b] Department of Pharmaceutical Sciences, Vanderbilt Ingram Cancer Center, Vanderbilt University Medical Center, 2220 Pierce Avenue, 777 Preston Research Building, Nashville, TN 37205, USA
* Corresponding author.
E-mail address: amanda.s.cass@vumc.org
Twitter: @HornLeora (L.H.); @amandacass (A.S.C.)

Thorac Surg Clin 30 (2020) 121–125
https://doi.org/10.1016/j.thorsurg.2020.01.011

starting to see oral small molecule inhibitors with promising efficacy. Immunohistochemical evaluation of PD-L1 also should be performed on all patients with advanced-stage disease regardless of histology. In patients who are both PD-L1 positive and harbor an actionable oncogenic driver, the presence of the mutation is considered more important in selection of therapy.

IMMUNOTHERAPY

Immune checkpoint inhibitors (ICIs) have been an important addition to the therapeutic armamentarium for patients with advanced NSCLC. Although promising results have been observed, these agents appear to have less efficacy in patients with driver mutations, such as EGR and ALK and in never smokers,[1,2] hence it is essential to perform mutational analysis before starting therapy in most circumstances. Food and Drug Administration (FDA) approval of ICI initially occurred in the second line (at time of progression after an initial course of chemotherapy) with nivolumab and atezolizumab approved regardless of PD-L1 expression, whereas pembrolizumab was approved only in patients with PD-L1 $\geq$1%.[3–5] The initial series of trials that led to these approvals demonstrated improved median overall survival (OS) and tolerability compared with single-agent docetaxel chemotherapy. Many early trials demonstrated an improvement in survival regardless of PD-L1 expression and, therefore, when ICIs were available only for patients who had progressed on platinum-based therapy many providers were not checking for PD-L1 expression and rather looking for response on imaging and in clinic.

Pembrolizumab is the only ICI currently approved as single-agent therapy in the first-line setting. This is based on results from the Keynote 024 trial, which was limited to patients with tumors that expressed PD-L1 of $\geq$ 50%.[6] The approval was subsequently expanded to include patients with tumors with PD-L1 greater than 1% based on similar results from the larger Keynote 042 trial.[7] Atezolizumab has also recently noted to have a significant improvement in OS for patients with high PD-L1 score compared with platinum-based chemotherapy.[8] All these trials showed significantly less toxicity in patients treated with an ICI compared with chemotherapy.

Several ICIs are now approved for use in combination with chemotherapy in patients with newly diagnosed stage IV disease, regardless of PD-L1 expression. Most trials evaluating these combinations excluded patients who were EGFR and ALK positive. In nonsquamous histology, pembrolizumab and atezolizumab are approved for use in combination with platinum-based therapy.[9,10] The only approved combination in the first-line setting for squamous cell NSCLC is pembrolizumab, which demonstrated superior response rate, progression-free survival (PFS), and OS, in combination with pembrolizumab, platinum, and taxane compared with platinum-taxane alone, and the benefits were seen regardless of PD-L1 expression.[11]

MOLECULAR TARGETED AGENTS

Patients with a tumor that harbors a mutation should receive targeted therapy directed to their mutation rather than cytotoxic chemotherapy or immunotherapy. These targeted therapies are associated with significant tumor regression as well as decreased toxicity compared with traditional cytotoxic therapy as discussed in the following sections.

EPIDERMAL GROWTH FACTOR RECEPTOR MUTATIONS

Erlotinib, gefitinib, afatinib, dacomitinib, and osimertinib are all EGFR tyrosine kinase inhibitors (TKIs) that are FDA approved for the treatment of patients with EGFR mutation–positive NSCLC. First-generation and second-generation EGFR inhibitors, erlotinib, gefitinib, and afatinib, have all shown increased PFS in patients with EGFR-mutated NSCLC when compared with chemotherapy.[12–14] Despite the observed survival benefits, most patients eventually develop therapeutic resistance.[12,15] Furthermore, approximately 50% of patients who develop acquired resistance to EGFR TKI therapy acquire a second-site mutation occurring within exon 20 (ie, T790M).[16,17] Osimertinib, the only third-generation EGFR inhibitor, was initially approved only for patients who develop an EGFR T790M mutation during a treatment with a first-generation or second-generation EGFR TKI.[18] Osimertinib has now been approved for first-line use based on results from FLAURA, a phase III, trial that compared osimertinib with erlotinib or gefitinib in the first-line setting for patients with EGFR-positive NSCLC. There were similar response rates in both groups, but osimertinib had prolonged PFS and OS. Osimertinib also demonstrated improved treatment of brain metastasis, an Achilles heel of first-generation and second-generation TKI agents.[19] Unavoidably, patients treated with osimertinib in the first-line setting will develop resistance, and understanding of these resistance mechanisms remains important. There are several ongoing trials that are examining these resistance mechanisms and looking at the most effective treatment strategies in patients at the time of progression.

ANAPLASTIC LYMPHOMA KINASE MUTATIONS

Crizotinib was the first FDA-approved ALK TKI based of the results of 2 phase III trials; PROFILE 1014 and 1007, which compared the TKI to standard-of-care chemotherapy in the first-line and recurrent setting. Both studies demonstrated an improvement in overall response rate and PFS with crizotinib compared with cytotoxic chemotherapy for patients with ALK-positive disease.[20–22] Similar to EGFR TKI therapy, patients treated with crizotinib will predictably develop resistance, with almost 50% of patients developing brain metastases at the time of progression. Later-generation ALK TKIs have been developed to overcome these resistance mechanisms, better penetrate the central nervous system (CNS), and improve side-effect profiles. Ceritinib was the first second-generation ALK TKI approved. It was initially approved for patients whose disease had progressed or who had proved intolerant to crizotinib,[23] and subsequently, ceritinib was approved in the first-line setting after head-to-head comparison with criztinib[24] Subsequently, 2 additional second-generation ALK TKIs were approved: alectinib was in the first line,[25] and brigatinib in second line.[26] Both agents have superior CNS penetration to crizotinib. Lorlatinib is a third-generation ALK TKI recently approved in patients with NSCLC who have progressed on prior ALK TKI.[27] Lorlatinib has a unique structure that maintains activity against the most common resistance mechanism, ALK G1202R.[27] The optimal sequencing of ALK TKIs has yet to be determined, but testing for resistance mechanisms at the time of progression is becoming increasingly important and can help guide therapy for second-line treatment with an oral agent rather than switching to chemotherapy.

RARE MUTATIONS

In addition to EGFR and ALK, several other targetable oncogenic drivers have been identified, including ROS-1, BRAF, NTRK, MET, RET, and HER-2. The discovery of these molecular mutations has caused a paradigm shift toward the discovery of agents to target these driver mutations. Structurally the ROS-1 oncogene is homologous to the ALK oncogene, which has been helpful in the discovery of agents targeting ROS-1.[28,29] Many of the ALK inhibitors also inhibit ROS-1. Currently, crizotinib and entrectinib are the only 2 FDA-approved therapies for patients with ROS-1 mutations.[30,31] A barrier to crizotinib treatment is the lack of CNS penetration, which is overcome by newer ROS-1 targeted agents, lorlatinib and entrectinib.[32]

A small proportion of NSCLCs can harbor a BRAF V600E mutation, most commonly seen in melanoma. Because of prior success in BRAF-mutated melanoma, 3 BRAF target regimens have been studied in NSCLC: vemurafenib, dabrafenib, and dabrafenib plus the MEK-inhibitor trametinib. NTRK mutations occur in a small percentage of patients with NSCLC, and there are 2 FDA-approved therapies for the treatment of patients with solid tumors that harbor an NTRK mutation: larotrectinib and entrectinib.[33,34] Although there are currently no FDA-approved therapies, there are several other driver mutations of interest in NSCLC, such as MET, RET, and HER-2, where there are commercially available agents approved for other molecular mutations that also improve survival for patients.

Molecular genotyping and the development of targeted agents to treat newly discovered molecular mutations has reinforced the heterogeneity and complexities of NSCLC, as well as the need for precision medicine to improve survival in these patients. Despite the progress that has been made, continued research is needed for more specific agents with less toxicity and better CNS penetration, as well as agents to treat patients who develop resistance against targeted treatments.

SUMMARY

The landscape of care in advanced NSCLC is rapidly progressing with previously unrecognized targets, new agents, and novel combinations being introduced and approved by the FDA on nearly a monthly basis. They provide improved survival for many, but responses are not universal, resistance continues to develop, and toxicity limits use in some. Large-panel molecular sequencing is becoming standard of care for nonsquamous histology because it guides personalized treatment decisions.

DISCLOSURE

L. Horn: Consulting AbbVie, Astra Zeneca, BMS, Merck, Pfizer, Xcovery, EMD Serono, Incyte, Roche-Genentech, Tessaro. Research funding: Boehringer Ingelheim, Xcovery, BMS. A. Cass: Consulting Roche-Genentech, Novartis.

REFERENCES

1. Kim JH, Kim HS, Kim BJ. Prognostic value of smoking status in non-small-cell lung cancer patients treated with immune checkpoint inhibitors: a meta-analysis. Oncotarget 2017;8:93149–55.
2. Gainor JF, Shaw AT, Sequist LV, et al. EGFR mutations and ALK rearrangements are associated with low response rates to PD-1 pathway blockade in non-small cell lung cancer: a retrospective analysis. Clin Cancer Res 2016;22: 4585–93.
3. Borghaei H, Paz-Ares L, Horn L, et al. Nivolumab versus Docetaxel in advanced nonsquamous non-small-cell lung cancer. N Engl J Med 2015;373: 1627–39.
4. Brahmer J, Reckamp KL, Baas P, et al. Nivolumab versus Docetaxel in advanced squamous-cell non-small-cell lung cancer. N Engl J Med 2015;373: 123–35.
5. Rizvi NA, Mazieres J, Planchard D, et al. Activity and safety of nivolumab, an anti-PD-1 immune checkpoint inhibitor, for patients with advanced, refractory squamous non-small-cell lung cancer (CheckMate 063): a phase 2, single-arm trial. Lancet Oncol 2015;16:257–65.
6. Reck M, Rodriguez-Abreu D, Robinson AG, et al. Pembrolizumab versus chemotherapy for PD-L1-positive non-small-cell lung cancer. N Engl J Med 2016;375:1823–33.
7. Mok TSK, Wu YL, Kudaba I, et al. Pembrolizumab versus chemotherapy for previously untreated, PD-L1-expressing, locally advanced or metastatic non-small-cell lung cancer (KEYNOTE-042): a randomised, open-label, controlled, phase 3 trial. Lancet 2019;393:1819–30.
8. Spigel D, de Marinis F, Giaccone G, et al. IMpower110: Interim overall survival (OS) analysis of a phase III study of atezolizumab (atezo) vs platinum-based chemotherapy (chemo) as first-line therapy. European Society of Medical Oncology Annual Meeting Barcelona, Spain, 27 September - 01 October, 2019..
9. Gandhi L, Rodriguez-Abreu D, Gadgeel S, et al. Pembrolizumab plus chemotherapy in metastatic non-small-cell lung cancer. N Engl J Med 2018; 378:2078–92.
10. Papadimitrakopoulou V, Cobo M, Bordoni R, et al. IMpower132: PFS and safety results with 1L Atezolizumab + Carboplatin/Cisplatin + Pemetrexed in Stage IV Non-Squamous NSCLC. World Conference on Lung Cancer. Toronto, Canada, September 23–26, 2018.
11. Paz-Ares L, Luft A, Vicente D, et al. Pembrolizumab plus chemotherapy for squamous non-small-cell lung cancer. N Engl J Med 2018;379: 2040–51.
12. Zhou C, Wu YL, Chen G, et al. Erlotinib versus chemotherapy as first-line treatment for patients with advanced EGFR mutation-positive non-small-cell lung cancer (OPTIMAL, CTONG-0802): a multicentre, open-label, randomised, phase 3 study. Lancet Oncol 2011;12:735–42.
13. Sequist LV, Yang JC, Yamamoto N, et al. Phase III study of afatinib or cisplatin plus pemetrexed in patients with metastatic lung adenocarcinoma with EGFR mutations. J Clin Oncol 2013;31:3327–34.
14. Maemondo M, Inoue A, Kobayashi K, et al. Gefitinib or chemotherapy for non-small-cell lung cancer with mutated EGFR. N Engl J Med 2010;362: 2380–8.
15. Riely GJ, Pao W, Pham D, et al. Clinical course of patients with non-small cell lung cancer and epidermal growth factor receptor exon 19 and exon 21 mutations treated with gefitinib or erlotinib. Clin Cancer Res 2006;12:839–44.
16. Kobayashi S, Boggon TJ, Dayaram T, et al. EGFR mutation and resistance of non-small-cell lung cancer to gefitinib. N Engl J Med 2005;352: 786–92.
17. Pao W, Miller VA, Politi KA, et al. Acquired resistance of lung adenocarcinomas to gefitinib or erlotinib is associated with a second mutation in the EGFR kinase domain. PLoS Med 2005;2:e73.
18. Mok TS, Wu YL, Ahn MJ, et al. Osimertinib or platinum-pemetrexed in EGFR T790M-positive lung cancer. N Engl J Med 2017;376:629–40.
19. Ramalingam SS, Vansteenkiste J, Planchard D, et al. Overall survival with osimertinib in untreated, EGFR-mutated advanced NSCLC. N Engl J Med 2020;382: 41–50.
20. Shaw AT, Kim DW, Nakagawa K, et al. Crizotinib versus chemotherapy in advanced ALK-positive lung cancer. N Engl J Med 2013;368:2385–94.
21. Solomon BJ, Mok T, Kim DW, et al. First-line crizotinib versus chemotherapy in ALK-positive lung cancer. N Engl J Med 2014;371:2167–77.
22. Solomon BJ, Kim DW, Wu YL, et al. Final overall survival analysis from a study comparing first-line crizotinib versus chemotherapy in ALK-mutation-positive non-small-cell lung cancer. J Clin Oncol 2018;36: 2251–8.
23. Shaw AT, Kim DW, Mehra R, et al. Ceritinib in ALK-rearranged non-small-cell lung cancer. N Engl J Med 2014;370:1189–97.
24. Soria JC, Tan DSW, Chiari R, et al. First-line ceritinib versus platinum-based chemotherapy in advanced ALK-rearranged non-small-cell lung cancer (ASCEND-4): a randomised, open-label, phase 3 study. Lancet 2017;389:917–29.
25. Peters S, Camidge DR, Shaw AT, et al. Alectinib versus Crizotinib in untreated ALK-positive non-small-cell lung cancer. N Engl J Med 2017;377: 829–38.

26. Kim DW, Tiseo M, Ahn MJ, et al. Brigatinib in patients with crizotinib-refractory anaplastic lymphoma kinase-positive non-small-cell lung cancer: a randomized, multicenter phase II trial. J Clin Oncol 2017;35:2490–8.
27. Shaw AT, Felip E, Bauer TM, et al. Lorlatinib in non-small-cell lung cancer with ALK or ROS1 rearrangement: an international, multicentre, open-label, single-arm first-in-man phase 1 trial. Lancet Oncol 2017;18:1590–9.
28. Stumpfova M, Jänne PA. Zeroing in on ROS1 rearrangements in non–small cell lung cancer. Clin Cancer Res 2012;18:4222–4.
29. Davies KD, Doebele RC. Molecular pathways: ROS1 fusion proteins in cancer. Clin Cancer Res 2013;19: 4040–5.
30. Shaw AT, Riely GJ, Bang Y-J, et al. Crizotinib in ROS1-rearranged advanced non-small-cell lung cancer (NSCLC): updated results, including overall survival, from PROFILE 1001. Ann Oncol 2019;30:1121–6.
31. Lin JJ, Shaw AT. Recent advances in targeting ROS1 in lung cancer. J Thorac Oncol 2019;12: 1611–25.
32. Doebele R, Ahn M, Siena S, et al. OA02.01 efficacy and safety of entrectinib in locally advanced or metastatic ROS1 fusion-positive non-small cell lung cancer. J Thorac Oncol 2018;13:S321–2.
33. Drilon A, Laetsch TW, Kummar S, et al. Efficacy of Larotrectinib in TRK fusion–positive cancers in adults and children. N Engl J Med 2018;378: 731–9.
34. Doebele R, Paz-Ares L, Farago AF, et al. Entrectinib in NTRK-fusion positive (NTRK-FP) non-small cell lung cancer (NSCLC): Integrated analysis of patients enrolled in three trials (STARTRK-2, STARTRK-1 and ALKA-372-001). Presented at: 2019 AACR Annual Meeting; March 29-April 3, 2019; Atlanta, GA. Abstract CT131.

Epidermal Growth Factor Receptor Mutations

Erin M. McLoughlin, MD[a], Ryan D. Gentzler, MD, MS[b,*]

KEYWORDS

• Non–small cell lung cancer • EGFR mutations • EGRF-TKIs • Erlotinib • Afatinib • Osimertinib
• Resistance mechanisms

KEY POINTS

- The identification and targeting of epidermal growth factor receptor (EGFR) mutations have been a paradigm shift in thoracic oncology and resulted in significant improvements in outcomes.
- Osimertinib is active against common EGFR mutations and the T790M resistance mutation and is considered standard of care in the first-line treatment of patients with advanced/metastatic non–small cell lung cancer (NSCLC).
- One of the main challenges in the treatment of EGFR-mutated lung cancer is the development of resistance to EGFR–tyrosine kinase inhibitors (TKIs), necessitating an urgent need to better understand mechanisms of resistance.
- EGFR-TKIs have been evaluated in earlier-stage disease as well as in combination with several other agents; however, at the current time, these approaches remain investigational.

BACKGROUND

The discovery of the epidermal growth factor receptor (EGFR) and development of targeted drugs have led to substantial gains in the treatment of non–small cell lung cancer (NSCLC). EGFR belongs to the HER/ErbB family of growth factor receptors. These receptors consist of an extracellular ligand binding domain, a transmember structure and an intracellular tyrosine kinase domain. When the EGFR extracellular domain binds one of its ligands, it forms a dimer with other EGFR and HER family members and activates several downstream pathways, resulting in increased cell proliferation and angiogenesis and a decrease in apoptosis.[1]

EGFR receptors are overexpressed in 40% to 80% of NSCLCs.[2] Despite high levels of EGFR protein expression, clinical responses to EGFR–tyrosine kinase inhibitors (TKIs) were observed in approximately only 10% to 18% of patients with chemorefractory disease.[3,4]

In 2004, Lynch and colleagues[5] identified 25 patients with clinically significant responses to gefitinib and a median duration of survival that exceeded 18 months. Gene sequencing in 9 patients revealed 8 had heterozygous mutations within the tyrosine kinase domain of EGFR, which activate the kinase domain and are sensitive to inhibition with gefitinib. Although the overexpression of EGFR in NSCLC was the biomarker that brought EGFR-TKIs into clinical use with early modest positive results, it is the identification and targeting of EGFR mutations that have been a paradigm shift in thoracic oncology.

Approximately 10% to 20% of lung adenocarcinomas in the United States and Europe and 40% to 50% in Asia have activating mutations of the tyrosine kinase domain of EGFR.[5–7] Exon 19 deletions and L858R point mutations account for 90%

[a] Division of Hematology/Oncology, University of Virginia School of Medicine, 1215 Lee Street, PO Box 800716, Charlottesville, VA 22908, USA; [b] Division of Hematology/Oncology, University of Virginia School of Medicine, PO Box 800716, Charlottesville, VA 22908, USA
* Corresponding author.
E-mail address: rg2uc@virginia.edu

Thorac Surg Clin 30 (2020) 127–136
https://doi.org/10.1016/j.thorsurg.2020.01.008

of the EGFR mutations and are highly predictive of response to EGFR-TKIs.[5,6]

DIAGNOSIS

The gold standard for diagnosis of EGFR-mutant lung cancer is direct DNA sequencing of tumor tissue DNA.

Tissue testing can be done as an individual EGFR test or as part of a larger panel of genes with next-generation sequencing technologies. Liquid biopsies, utilizing various nucleic acid sequencing methods to identify mutations in circulating tumor DNA, are becoming more frequently utilized. This method is appealing when tissue is insufficient or when obtaining additional tissue is impractical. Collectively, these methods have excellent specificity and patient outcomes are similar whether mutations are detected via tissue or circulating tumor DNA.[8,9] The sensitivity is reported to be approximately 80%; therefore, negative tests should be interpreted with some caution.[10]

TREATMENT

Epidermal Growth Factor Receptor–Tyrosine Kinase Inhibitors for Advanced/Metastatic Disease

Multiple phase III trials of EGFR-TKIs have improved radiographic response and progression-free survival (PFS) for patients with EGFR mutations in the first-line metastatic setting compared with chemotherapy. Newer-generation TKIs have improved on the gains seen with first-generation EGFR-TKIs (**Table 1**).[11–15] EGFR-TKIs have reduced toxic effects and perform better with respect to quality-of-life measures.

Despite the current standard approach to use EGFR-TKIs in EGFR-mutated patients, earlier trials identified a benefit in an unselected population of patients with NSCLC. Gefitinib demonstrated improved response rates in the third-line setting for unselected NSCLC patients who had progressed through 2 lines of chemotherapy and initially was granted accelerated Food and Drug Administration (FDA) approval.[16] Erlotinib was approved the following year based on the BR.21 trial that showed improved PFS and OS (6.7 months vs 4.7 months: hazard ratio [HR] 0.7; *P*<.001).[17] Later, the phase III trial, ISEL, comparing gefitinib to placebo failed to replicate a survival benefit in a similar population, and gefitinib lost its FDA approval but continued to be used outside of the United States.[18] It was not until more than 10 years later that gefitinib was granted approval status in the United States and erlotinib's approval was restricted to patients whose tumors possessed an EGFR mutation.

Although early trials identified certain clinical characteristics (ie, female smokers and never smokers) of patients who derived the greatest benefits, it is now known that the presence of specific EGFR mutations are a more robust predictor of response to EGFR-TKIs. In the IPASS trial, overall response rates (ORRs) for patients with and without an EGFR mutation who received gefitinib were 71.2% versus 1.1%, respectively.[11] Subgroup analysis showed gefitinib was beneficial for EGFR-positive patients (HR 0.48; *P*<.001) but was detrimental for those without mutations (HR 2.85; *P*<.001) compared with chemotherapy.[11] This PFS benefit was demonstrated in multiple prospective phase III trials comparing EGFR-TKIs with chemotherapy.[12–15] With longer follow-up, first-generation EGFR-TKIs have not demonstrated a survival benefit, largely attributed to the crossover design of these studies, which allowed patients on the control arm to eventually get the more effective therapy.[19–23]

The second generation EGFR-TKIs, afatinib and dacomitinib, irreversibly bind to the tyrosine kinase of EGFR and other ErbB family members and are approved in the front-line metastatic setting based on demonstrated improvements in PFS in several large phase III trials (see **Table 1**).[24–26] Survival data from ARCHER 1050, which compared first-line dacomitinib to gefitinib, showed a median overall survival (OS) of 34.1 months with dacomitinib, compared with 26.8 months in the gefitinib arm, representing a more than 7-month improvement in survival, albeit with more grade 3 toxicities reported in patients receiving dacomitinib.[27]

Osimertinib, a third-generation, irreversible EGFR-TKI, inhibits common EGFR mutations as well as the T790M resistance mutation. FLAURA evaluated osimertinib in the first-line setting compared with first-generation EGFR-TKIs; 556 patients with EGFR-positive advanced NSCLC were randomized to osimertinib versus investigator choice of erlotinib or gefitinib.[28] The primary endpoint of PFS was significantly longer with osimertinib (18.9 months vs 10 months; HR 0.46; *P*<.001). These results were practice changing and osimertinib is now the preferred first-line agent for EGFR mutation–positive NSCLC. OS was immature at last report of trial data, but a press release in August 2019 indicates the trial met its secondary endpoint of OS.[29]

Does mutation type matter?

A combined planned analysis from LUX-Lung 3 (afatinib vs cisplatin/pemetrexed) and LUX-Lung 6 (afatinib vs cisplatin/gemcitabine) showed afatinib did not improve OS.[30] OS was improved, however, with afatinib for the subgroups of patients

Table 1
Select first-line phase III trials for advanced/metastatic disease

Study	Epidermal Growth Factor Receptor Status	N	Primary Outcome	Design	Outcomes
IPASS, 11 Asia, 2009	EGFR unselected	1217 EGFR+ positive= 261	PFS	Gefitinib vs carboplatin + paclitaxel	12-mo PFS, 24.9% (gefitinib) vs 6.7% (HR 0.74; *P*<.001) Subgroup EGFR-positive (HR 0.48; *P*<.001) Updated survival:[19] OS (HR 0.90; *P* = .109) Subgroup EGFR mutation–positive (HR 1.00; *P* = .990)
EURTAC,[15] Europe, 2012	EGFR selected	173	PFS	Erlotinib vs cisplatin + docetaxel or gemcitabine	Median PFS 9.7 mo (erlotinib) vs 5.2 mo (HR 0.37; *P*<.0001) Updated survival:[23] 22.9 mo (erlotinib) vs 19.6 mo (HR OS was 0.92; *P* = .68)
LUX-Lung 3,[24] Europe, North and South America, and Australia, 2013	EGFR selected	345	PFS	Afatinib vs cisplatin + pemetrexed	Exon 19 del and L858R EGFR mutations, n = 308 Median PFS 13.6 mo (afatinib) vs 6.9 mo (HR 0.47; *P* = .001) Updated survival:[30] 28. 2 mo (afatinib) vs 28.2 mo (HR 0.88; *P* = .39) Subgroup exon 19 deletion: 33.3 mo (afatinib) vs 21.1 mo (HR 0.54; *P* = .0015)
LUX-Lung 6,[25] Asia, 2014	EGFR selected	364	PFS	Afatinib vs cisplatin + gemcitabine	Median PFS was 11.0 mo (afatinib) vs 5.6 mo (HR 0.28; *P*<.0001) Updated survival:[30] 23.1 mo (afatinib) vs 23.5 mo (HR 0.93; *P* = .61) Subgroup exon 19 deletion: 31.4 mo (afatinib) vs 18.4 mo (HR 0.64; *P* = .023)

(*continued on next page*)

Table 1
(*continued*)

Study	Epidermal Growth Factor Receptor Status	N	Primary Outcome	Design	Outcomes
ARCHER 1050,[26] 2017	EGFR selected	452	PFS	Dacomitinib vs gefitinib	Median PFS 14.7 mo (dacomitinib) vs 9.2 mo (gefitinib) (HR 0.59; $P<.0001$) Updated survival:[27] Median OS 34.1 mo (dacomitinib) vs 26.8 mo (gefitinib) (HR OS 0.760; $P = .0438$)
FLAURA,[28] 2018	EGFR selected	556	PFS	Osimertinib vs standard TKI (erlotinib or gefitinib)	Median PFS 18.9 mo (osimertinib) vs 10.2 mo (standard TKI) (HR disease progression or death 0.46; $P<.001$) Updated survival:[29] improved OS with osimertinib vs standard TKI

with exon 19 deletions in both trials. An association with improved PFS in patients with exon 19 deletion mutations was observed in several first-generation TKI studies, including IPASS (HR 0.38 for del19 vs HR 0.55 for L858R)[19] and EURTAC (HR 0.30 del19 vs 0.55 for L858R).[15] but were not statistically significant.

Although exon 19 deletions and L858R point mutations account for 90% of mutations, several other mutations, including G719X, L861Q, S7681, EGFR fusions, and exon 20 insertions, have been reported but show variable response to TKIs.[31] The G719X mutations are sensitizing mutations, whereas the exon 20 insertions and de novo T790M mutations typically are resistant to first-generation and second-generation EGFR-TKIs.

Exon 20 mutations confer a poor response to EGFR-TKIs but efforts to treat this subgroup are ongoing. TAK-788 and poziotinib are investigational EGFR/HER2 inhibitors with antitumor activity in this population.[32,33] In addition, there are preclinical data and a case report to indicate osimertinib, at a dose of 180 mg, may be able to overcome this inherent resistance, and a clinical trial is ongoing.[34,35]

Dealing with resistance

Resistance to first-generation and second-generation EGFR-TKIs typically develops within 9 months to 14 months.[11–15,24–26] EGFR pThr790Met (T790M) point mutations are identified in greater than 50% of patients who develop disease progression on first-line TKIs.[36,37] Other mechanisms of resistance have been identified, including mutations in PIKC3 and BRAF, small cell transformation, and amplification of HER2, MET, and MAPK1.[38]

Osimertinib is active against common EGFR mutations and the T790M resistance mutation. In AURA3, osimertinib was compared with carboplatin/pemetrexed in T790M-positive patients with disease progression after first-line EGFR-TKI therapy.[39] PFS was significantly longer with osimertinib compared with chemotherapy (10.1 months vs 4.4 months, respectively; HR 0.41; *P*<.001). In patients with central nervous system metastases, a population with an overall worse prognosis, PFS was longer, at 8.5 months versus 4.2 months, respectively, in the chemotherapy arm (HR 0.32).[39]

Efforts to characterize mechanisms of resistance to osimertinib are ongoing, but reports to date have demonstrated a heterogeneous group of mechanisms, including acquired EGFR mutations, predominantly C797; off-target mutations; rearrangements; fusions; and transformation to squamous or small cell lung cancer.[40,41] Targeting mutations or rearrangements involving RET, ALK, and BRAF have been reported with some success in case reports.[42,43]

Combination Therapy in the Advanced/Metastatic Setting

In efforts to overcome resistance to EGFR-TKIs or improve on single-agent activity in the first-line setting, several combinations have been studied.

Epidermal growth factor receptor–tyrosine kinase inhibitors plus epidermal growth factor receptor monoclonal antibodies

Preclinical data that combination afatinib and cetuximab could overcome resistance mediated by the acquired T790M mutation provided the rationale for a phase Ib trial of 126 patients with acquired resistance to erlotinib or gefitinib. An ORR of 29% was observed.[44] This study enrolled patients regardless of T790M status and there were no significant differences in response based on T790M status. Incidence rates of adverse events were high (94% all grades and 50% grades 3/4). Osimertinib has largely replaced this regimen due to better efficacy and tolerability for patients with acquired T790M mutations. For patients with non–T790-acquired resistance, this could be considered, given the responses seen in the T790M-negative population.

Epidermal growth factor receptor–tyrosine kinase inhibitors plus chemotherapy

Studies evaluating combination chemotherapy and EGFR-TKIs were first conducted in unselected populations with no known EGFR mutations. SATURN was a phase III trial of maintenance erlotinib after chemotherapy that showed a statistically significant 1-month OS improvement with erlotinib maintenance.[45] Prospective molecular analysis identified the magnitude of benefit was far greater among patients with EGFR mutations (PFS 44.6 months with erlotinib vs PFS 13.0 months with placebo) than those without EGFR mutations (PFS 12.0 months with erlotinib vs PFS 8.9 months with placebo).[46]

Two studies in patients with known EGFR mutations have shown promising results combining gefitinib with carboplatin and with pemetrexed. A phase III Japanese trial (NEJ009) evaluating gefitinib plus chemotherapy versus gefitinib alone demonstrated an improvement in PFS (20.9 months vs 11.2 months, respectively; HR 0.493; *P*<.001) and OS (52.2 months vs 38.8 months, respectively; *P* = .013).[47] Similar improvements in PFS and OS were seen in a randomized phase III study from Tata Memorial Hospital in Mumbai, India.[48] Given advances with osimertinib in the FLAURA trial, it is unclear how this combination compares to osimertinib alone or osimertinib plus chemotherapy. FLAURA2 will compare osimertinib alone versus osimertinib plus platinum-based chemotherapy in the front-line setting for locally advanced/metastatic EGFR-mutated NSCLC.

Epidermal growth factor receptor–tyrosine kinase inhibitors plus anti–vascular endothelial growth factor agents

Combination of vascular endothelial growth factor (VEGF) monoclonal antibodies with EGFR-TKIs is an appealing strategy based on the JO25567 phase 2 trial, which showed that the addition of bevacizumab to erlotinib in EGFR-mutant patients improved PFS (16.0 months vs 9.7 months without bevacizumab; HR 0.54; P = 0.0015).[49] The NEJ026 study, with similar design, showed an improved PFS with erlotinib and bevacizumab (16.9 months vs 13.3 months without bevacizumab) in an interim analysis (HR 0.605; *P* = .0157).[50] Preliminary results of an ongoing phase 1/2 study of 49 patients treated with osimertinib and bevacizumab reported an ORR of 69% and HR for 12-month PFS of 0.70 (95% CI, 0.57–0.84).[51] TORG1833 is a similar ongoing phase 2 trial evaluating osimertinib in combination with ramucirumab, a monoclonal antibody targeted against the VEGF-receptor (VEGFR2).[52] RELAY, a phase 3 trial, is randomizing patients with metastatic EGFR-mutant patients to erlotinib in combination with ramucirumab versus placebo.[53] Preliminary results reported at American Society of Clinical Oncology 2019 annual meeting demonstrated dual blockade led to an improvement in PFS compared with erlotinib plus placebo (19.4 months vs 12.4 months, respectively; HR 0.591; *P*<.0001). Final results from these trials are awaited.

Immunotherapy for epidermal growth factor receptor–mutant non–small cell lung cancer

A meta-analysis, including CheckMate 057 (nivolumab), Keynote-0.001 (pembrolizumab), POPLAR, and OAK (atezolizumab), which all compared immunotherapy to docetaxel in previously treated patients, concluded that immune checkpoint inhibitors do not improve OS in patients with EGFR-mutant lung cancer.[54] In a subgroup analysis from IMpower 150, the 91 patients with EGFR mutations maintained an OS improvement with the addition of atezolizumab to bevacizumab and chemotherapy, suggesting this combination may be able to overcome the lack of benefit seen with immunotherapy in other trials.[55] Further studies are needed to determine the role of immunotherapy in this disease.

Earlier-stage Disease

Despite complete surgical resection, approximately 30% to 55% of patients with NSCLC develop disease recurrence after surgery.[56] Cisplatin-based chemotherapy has improved survival for patients with stages IIA–IIIA disease (stage IB >4 cm is now categorized as stage IIA in the *AJCC Cancer Staging Manual*,[57] eighth edition).[58,59] Given significant efficacy of EGFR-TKIs over chemotherapy in the metastatic setting, there has been interest in evaluating EGFR inhibitors in earlier-stage disease. Three large phase 3 trials have evaluated their use in the adjuvant setting.

As in the metastatic setting, earlier adjuvant EGFR-TKI trials enrolled unselected patients. EGFR mutation subgroup analysis from RADIANT, a phase 3 trial that compared 24 months of erlotinib to placebo in patients with resected stages IB–IIIA NSCLC, showed improved disease-free survival (DFS).[60] Due to hierarchical testing, this was not statistically significant and survival curves overlapped by 48 months. This trial did not meet its DFS and OS endpoints in the entire trial population of patients who were selected only for EGFR overexpression.

SELECT, a single-arm phase 2 trial of EGFR-mutant stages IA–IIIA patients, evaluated 2 years of adjuvant erlotinib after standard adjuvant chemotherapy. The median DFS and OS have not been reached, but 5-year OS is 86%, an improvement based on historical controls.[61] A majority of patients with recurrence (26/40) were retreated with erlotinib for a median duration of 13 months.

ADJUVANT and EVAN were phase 3 trials that randomized completely resected patients with EGFR mutations to gefitinib and erlotinib, respectively, versus chemotherapy. ADJUVANT enrolled patients with stages II–IIIA disease and EVAN enrolled only patients with stage IIIA disease.[62,63] Both studies demonstrated improved DFS with the EGFR-TKI, but OS data are immature. A meta-analysis, including ADJUVANT and EVAN, showed a statistically significant improvement in 5-year OS (HR 0.48).[64]

Neoadjuvant EGFR-TKIs also have been evaluated. EMERGING/CTONG 1103, an ongoing phase 2 trial comparing erlotinib to chemotherapy in stage IIIA-N2 EGFR mutation–positive NSCLC, recently reported an improvement in PFS with erlotinib compared with chemotherapy

(21.5 months vs 11.9 months, respectively; HR 0.42; $P = .0003$).[65]

Despite earlier negative trials in an unselected NSCLC population, there has been renewed interest given positive findings from more recent trials for patients with EGFR mutations. Larger studies are needed to determine the optimal sequencing and potential benefit of EGFR targeted therapy in this setting. In the United States, the ALCHEMIST EGFR study (NCT02193282) is a phase 3 randomized trial evaluating adjuvant erlotinib versus observation for patients with surgically resected stages IB (>4 cm)–IIIA (*AJCC Cancer Staging Manual*,[66] seventh edition) after completion of standard adjuvant chemotherapy. It remains unclear whether this strategy ultimately can improve long-term survival or cure rates for patients with earlier-stage disease.

SUMMARY

- The identification of EGFR sensitizing mutations and the development of targeted EGFR-TKIs have transformed the way EGFR-mutant lung cancer is treated and drastically improved on the previous standard.
- Osimertinib currently is considered the standard of care for the treatment of metastatic disease.
- Given the successes of TKIs in the metastatic setting, efforts are ongoing to incorporate them into the treatment paradigm for earlier-stage disease, but chemotherapy remains the standard adjuvant therapy at this time.
- Ongoing efforts to combine TKIs with other modalities offer promise; however, there is an urgent need to better understand the mechanisms of acquired resistance because chemotherapy remains the standard second line after disease progression on osimertinib.

DISCLOSURE

Dr E.M. McLoughlin has nothing to disclose. Dr R.D. Gentzler has the following disclosures in the past 3 years: personal fees outside the submitted work from Merck, Takeda, Pfizer AstraZeneca, and Bristol Myers Squibb and research funding to his institution from Merck, Takeda, Pfizer Helsinn, and Bristol Myers Squibb.

REFERENCES

1. Seshacharyulu P, Ponnusamy MP, Haridas D, et al. Expert opinion on therapeutic targets targeting the EGFR signaling pathway in cancer therapy targeting the EGFR signaling pathway in cancer therapy. Expert Opin Ther Targets 2017. https://doi.org/10.1517/14728222.2011.648617.
2. Gupta R, Dastane AM, Forozan F, et al. Evaluation of EGFR abnormalities in patients with pulmonary adenocarcinoma: the need to test neoplasms with more than one method. Mod Pathol 2009. https://doi.org/10.1038/modpathol.2008.182.
3. Kris MG, Natale RB, Herbst RS, et al. Efficacy of gefitinib, an inhibitor of the epidermal growth factor receptor tyrosine kinase, in symptomatic patients with NSCLC: a randomized trial. J Am Med Assoc 2003. https://doi.org/10.1001/jama.290.16.2149.
4. Fukuoka M, Yano S, Giaccone G, et al. Multi-institutional randomized phase II trial of gefitinib for previously treated patients with advanced NSCLC (The IDEAL1 Trial) [corrected] [Erratum appears in J Clin Oncol. 2004;22(23):4811]. J Clin Oncol 2003; 21(12):2237–46.
5. Lynch TJ, Bell DW, Sordella R, et al. Activating mutations in the epidermal growth factor receptor underlying responsiveness of NSCLC to gefitinib. N Engl J Med 2004. https://doi.org/10.1056/nejmoa040938.
6. Paez JG, Jänne PA, Lee JC, et al. EGFR mutations in lung, cancer: correlation with clinical response to gefitinib therapy. Science 2004;80. https://doi.org/10.1126/science.1099314.
7. Li T, Kung HJ, Mack PC, et al. Genotyping and genomic profiling of NSCLC: implications for current and future therapies. J Clin Oncol 2013. https://doi.org/10.1200/JCO.2012.45.3753.
8. Qiu M, Wang J, Xu Y, et al. Circulating tumor DNA is effective for the detection of EGFR mutation in NSCLC: a meta-analysis. Cancer Epidemiol Biomarkers Prev 2015. https://doi.org/10.1158/1055-9965.EPI-14-0895.
9. Passiglia F, Rizzo S, Di Maio M, et al. The diagnostic accuracy of circulating tumor DNA for the detection of EGFR-T790M mutation in NSCLC: a systematic review and meta-analysis. Sci Rep 2018;8(1):13379.
10. Thompson JC, Yee SS, Troxel AB, et al. Detection of therapeutically targetable driver and resistance mutations in lung cancer patients by next-generation sequencing of cell-free circulating tumor DNA. Clin Cancer Res 2016;22(23):5772–82.
11. Mok TS, Wu Y-L, Thongprasert S, et al. Gefitinib or carboplatin–paclitaxel in pulmonary adenocarcinoma. N Engl J Med 2009. https://doi.org/10.1056/nejmoa0810699.
12. Mitsudomi T, Morita S, Yatabe Y, et al. Gefitinib versus cisplatin plus docetaxel in patients with NSCLC harbouring mutations of the epidermal growth factor receptor (WJTOG3405): an open label, randomised phase 3 trial. Lancet Oncol 2010. https://doi.org/10.1016/S1470-2045(09)70364-X.
13. Maemondo M, Inoue A, Kobayashi K, et al. Gefitinib or chemotherapy for non-small-cell lung cancer with

mutated EGFR. N Engl J Med 2010. https://doi.org/10.1056/NEJMoa0909530.
14. Zhou S, Ren S, Ye M, et al. Erlotinib versus chemotherapy as first-line treatment for patients with advanced EGFR mutation-positive non-small-cell lung cancer (OPTIMAL, CTONG-0802): a multicentre, open-label, randomised, phase 3 study. Lancet Oncol 2011. https://doi.org/10.1016/s1470-2045(11)70184-x.
15. Rosell R, Carcereny E, Gervais R, et al. Erlotinib versus standard chemotherapy as first-line treatment for European patients with advanced EGFR mutation-positive non-small-cell lung cancer (EURTAC): a multicentre, open-label, randomised phase 3 trial. Lancet Oncol 2012. https://doi.org/10.1016/S1470-2045(11)70393-X.
16. Cohen MH. FDA drug approval summary: gefitinib (ZD1839) (Iressa(R)) tablets. Oncologist 2003;8(4):303–6.
17. Shepherd FA, Rodrigues Pereira J, Ciuleanu T, et al. Erlotinib in previously treated non–small-cell lung cancer. N Engl J Med 2005. https://doi.org/10.1056/nejmoa050753.
18. Thatcher N, Chang A, Parikh P, et al. Gefitinib plus best supportive care in previously treated patients with refractory advanced non-small-cell lung cancer: results from a randomised, placebo-controlled, multicentre study (Iressa Survival Evaluation in Lung Cancer). Lancet 2005. https://doi.org/10.1016/S0140-6736(05)67625-8.
19. Fukuoka M, Wu YL, Thromgprasert S, et al. Biomarker analyses and final overall survival results from a phase III, randomized, open-label, first-line study of gefitinib versus carboplatin/paclitaxel in clinically selected patients with advanced NSCLC in Asia (IPASS). J Clin Oncol 2011. https://doi.org/10.1200/JCO.2010.33.4235.
20. Inoue A, Kobayashi K, Maemondo M, et al. Updated overall survival results from a randomized phase III trial comparing gefitinib with carboplatin-paclitaxel for chemo-naïve non-small cell lung cancer with sensitive EGFR gene mutations (NEJ002). Ann Oncol 2013. https://doi.org/10.1093/annonc/mds214.
21. Mitsudomi T, Morita S, Yatabe Y, et al. Updated overall survival results of WJTOG 3405, a randomized phase III trial comparing gefitinib (G) with cisplatin plus docetaxel (CD) as the first-line treatment for patients with NSCLC harboring mutations of the epidermal growth factor receptor (EGFR). J Clin Oncol 2012;30(15_supp):7521.
22. Zhou C, Wu YL, Liu X, et al. Overall survival (OS) results from OPTIMAL (CTONG0802), a phase III trial of erlotinib (E) versus carboplatin plus gemcitabine (GC) as first-line treatment for Chinese patients with EGFR mutation-positive advanced NSCLC. J Clin Oncol 2012;30(15_suppl):7520.
23. Leon LF, Golsorkhi A, Liu S, et al. Overall survival analyses of first-line erlotinib versus chemotherapy in the EURTAC study population controlling for the use of post-study therapy. Ann Oncol 2014; 25(suppl_4). https://doi.org/10.1093/annonc/mdu349.
24. Sequist LV, Yang JCH, Yamamoto N, et al. Phase III study of afatinib or cisplatin plus pemetrexed in patients with metastatic lung adenocarcinoma with EGFR mutations. J Clin Oncol 2013. https://doi.org/10.1200/JCO.2012.44.2806.
25. Wu YL, Zhou C, Hu CP, et al. Afatinib versus cisplatin plus gemcitabine for first-line treatment of Asian patients with advanced NSCLC harbouring EGFR mutations (LUX-Lung 6): an open-label, randomised phase 3 trial. Lancet Oncol 2014. https://doi.org/10.1016/S1470-2045(13)70604-1.
26. Wu YL, Cheng Y, Zhou X, et al. Dacomitinib versus gefitinib as first-line treatment for patients with EGFR-mutation-positive non-small-cell lung cancer (ARCHER 1050): a randomised, open-label, phase 3 trial. Lancet Oncol 2017. https://doi.org/10.1016/S1470-2045(17)30608-3.
27. Mok TS, Cheng Y, Zhou X, et al. Improvement in overall survival in a randomized study that compared dacomitinib with gefitinib in patients with advanced non–small-cell lung cancer and EGFR -activating mutations. J Clin Oncol 2018. https://doi.org/10.1200/jco.2018.78.7994.
28. Soria J-C, Ohe Y, Vansteenkiste J, et al. Osimertinib in untreated EGFR -mutated advanced NSCLC. N Engl J Med 2017. https://doi.org/10.1056/nejmoa1713137.
29. Kemp A. Tagrisso significantly improves overall survival in the Phase III FLAURA trial for 1st-line EGFR-mutated NSCLC. Available at: https://www.astrazeneca.com/media-centre/press-releases/2019/tagrisso-significantly-improves-overall-survival-in-the-phase-iii-flaura-trial-for-1st-line-egfr-mutated-non-small-cell-lung-cancer-09082019.html. Accessed February 9, 2020.
30. Yang JCH, Wu YL, Schuler M, et al. Afatinib versus cisplatin-based chemotherapy for EGFR mutation-positive lung adenocarcinoma (LUX-Lung 3 and LUX-Lung 6): analysis of overall survival data from two randomised, phase 3 trials. Lancet Oncol 2015. https://doi.org/10.1016/S1470-2045(14)71173-8.
31. Westover D, Zugazagoitia J, Cho BC, et al. Mechanisms of acquired resistance to first-and second-generation EGFR tyrosine kinase inhibitors. Ann Oncol 2018. https://doi.org/10.1093/annonc/mdx703.
32. Janne PA, Neal JW, Camidge R, et al. Antitumor activity of TAK-788 in NSCLC with EGFR exon 20 insertions. J Clin Oncol 2019;37(suppl) [abstract: 9007].

33. Heymach J J, Negrao M, Robichaux J, et al. A phase II trial of poziotinib in EGFR and HER2 exon 20 mutant NSCLC. J Thorac Oncol 2018;13(10):S323–4.
34. Riess J, Floch N, Martin M, et al. Antitumor activity of osimertinib in NSCLC harboring EGFR exon 20 insertions. J Clin Oncol 2017;35(15_suppl).
35. Piotrowska Z, Fintelmann FJ, Sequist LV, et al. Response to osimertinib in an EGFR exon 20 insertion-positive lung adenocarcinoma. J Thorac Oncol 2018;13(10):e204–6.
36. Oxnard GR, Arcila ME, Sima CS, et al. Acquired resistance to EGFR tyrosine kinase inhibitors in EGFR-mutant lung cancer: distinct natural history of patients with tumors harboring the T790M mutation. Clin Cancer Res 2011;17(6):1616–22.
37. Yu HA, Arcila ME, Rekhtman N, et al. Analysis of tumor specimens at the time of acquired resistance to EGFR-TKI therapy in 155 patients with EGFR-mutant lung cancers. Clin Cancer Res 2013. https://doi.org/10.1158/1078-0432.CCR-12-2246.
38. Stewart EK, Tan SZ, Liu G, et al. Known and putative mechanisms of resistance to EGFR targeted therapies in NSCLC patients with EGFR mutations-a review. Transl Lung Cancer Res 2015. https://doi.org/10.3978/j.issn.2218-6751.2014.11.06.
39. Mok TS, Wu Y-L, Ahn M-J, et al. Osimertinib or platinum–pemetrexed in EGFR T790M–positive lung cancer. N Engl J Med 2016. https://doi.org/10.1056/nejmoa1612674.
40. Oxnard GR, Hu Y, Mileham KF, et al. Assessment of resistance mechanisms and clinical implications in patients with EGFR T790M-positive lung cancer and acquired resistance to osimertinib. JAMA Oncol 2018;4(11):1527–34.
41. Schoenfeld AJ, Chan JM, Rizvi H, et al. Tissue-based molecular and histological landscape of acquired resistance to osimertinib given initially or at relapse in patients with EGFR-mutant lung cancers. J Clin Oncol 2019;37(suppl) [abstract: 9028].
42. Offin M, Somwar R, Rekhtman N, et al. Acquired ALK and RET gene fusions as mechanisms of resistance to osimertinib in EGFR -mutant lung cancers. JCO Precis Oncol 2018;(2):1–12.
43. Piotrowska Z, Isozaki H, Lennerz JK, et al. Landscape of acquired resistance to osimertinib in EGFR-mutant NSCLC and clinical validation of combined EGFR and RET inhibition with osimertinib and BLU-667 for acquired RET fusion. Cancer Discov 2018;8(12):1529–39.
44. Janjigian YY, Smit EF, Groen HJM, et al. Dual inhibition of EGFR with afatinib and cetuximab in kinase inhibitor-resistant EGFR-mutant lung cancer with and without T790M mutations. Cancer Discov 2014;4(9):1036–45.
45. Cappuzzo F, Ciuleanu T, Stelmakh L, et al. Erlotinib as maintenance treatment in advanced non-small-cell lung cancer: a multicentre, randomised, placebo-controlled phase 3 study. Lancet Oncol 2010. https://doi.org/10.1016/S1470-2045(10)70112-1.
46. Brugger W, Triller N, Blasinska-Morawiec M, et al. Prospective molecular marker analyses of EGFR and KRAS from a randomized, placebo-controlled study of erlotinib maintenance therapy in advanced non-small-cell lung cancer. J Clin Oncol 2011. https://doi.org/10.1200/JCO.2010.31.8162.
47. Nakamura A, Inoue A, Morita S, et al. Phase III study comparing gefitinib monotherapy (G) to combination therapy with gefitinib, carboplatin, and pemetrexed (GCP) for untreated patients (pts) with advanced non-small cell lung cancer (NSCLC) with EGFR mutations (NEJ009). J Clin Oncol 2018;36(15_suppl): 9005.
48. Noronha V, Patil VM, joshi a, et al. gefitinib versus gefitinib plus pemetrexed and carboplatin chemotherapy in EGFR-mutated lung cancer. J Clin Oncol 2019;37(15):9001.
49. Seto T, Kato T, Nishio M, et al. Erlotinib alone or with bevacizumab as first-line therapy in patients with advanced non-squamous non-small-cell lung cancer harbouring EGFR mutations (JO25567): an open-label, randomised, multicentre, phase 2 study. Lancet Oncol 2014;15(11):1236–44.
50. Saito H, Fukuhara T, Furuya N, et al. Erlotinib plus bevacizumab versus erlotinib alone in patients with EGFR-positive advanced non-squamous non-small-cell lung cancer (NEJ026): interim analysis of an open-label, randomised, multicentre, phase 3 trial. Lancet Oncol 2019. https://doi.org/10.1016/S1470-2045(19)30035-X.
51. Yu HA, Kim R, Makhnin A, et al. A phase 1/2 study of osimertinib and bevacizumab as initial treatment for patients with metastatic EGFR-mutant lung cancers. J Clin Oncol 2019;37(suppl) [abstract: 9086].
52. Nakahara Y, Kato T, Isomura R, et al. A multicenter, open label, randomized phase II study of osimertinib plus ramucirumab versus osimertinib alone as initial chemotherapy for EGFR mutation-positive non-squamous non-small cell lung cancer: TORG1833. J Clin Oncol 2019;37 [abstract: TPS9120].
53. Nakagawa K, Garon EB, Set T, et al. RELAY: a multinational, double-blind, randomized Phase 3 study of erlotinib (ERL) in combination with ramucirumab (RAM) or placebo (PL) in previously untreated patients with epidermal growth factor receptor mutation-positive (EGFRm) metastatic NSCLC. J Clin Oncol 2019;37(suppl) [abstract: 9000].
54. Lee CK, Man J, Lord S, et al. Checkpoint inhibitors in metastatic EGFR-mutated NSCLC —a meta-analysis. J Thorac Oncol 2017. https://doi.org/10.1016/j.jtho.2016.10.007.
55. Reck M, Mok TSK, Nishio M, et al. Atezolizumab plus bevacizumab and chemotherapy in NSCLC (IMpower150): key subgroup analyses of patients with

EGFR mutations or baseline liver metastases in a randomised, open-label phase 3 trial. Lancet Respir Med 2019. https://doi.org/10.1016/S2213-2600(19)30084-0.
56. Taylor MD, Nagji AS, Bhamidipati CM, et al. Tumor recurrence after complete resection for NSCLC. Ann Thorac Surg 2012;93(6):1813–20 [discussion: 1820–1].
57. Available at: https://www.amazon.com/AJCC-Cancer-Staging-Manual-Mahul/dp/3319406175/ref=sr_1_1?gclid=EAIaIQobChMI1J6NyPrF5wIVCZyzCh1KUwKSEAAYASAAEgITy_D_BwE&hvadid=345573984463&hvdev=c&hvlocphy=9008341&hvnetw=g&hvpos=1t1&hvqmt=e&hvrand=15196786613092524843&hvtargid=kwd-733802856676&hydadcr=20837_10175449&keywords=ajcc+cancer+staging+manual+8th+ed&qid=1581302433&sr=8-1.
58. NSCLC Meta-analyses Collaborative Group, Arriagada R, Auperin A, Burdett S, et al. Adjuvant chemotherapy, with or without postoperative radiotherapy, in operable non-small-cell lung cancer: two meta-analyses of individual patient data. Lancet 2010;375(9722):1267–77.
59. Pignon JP, Tribodet H, Scagliotti GV, et al. Lung adjuvant cisplatin evaluation: a pooled analysis by the LACE collaborative group. J Clin Oncol 2008; 26(21):3552–9.
60. Kelly K, Altorki NK, Eberhardt WEE, et al. Adjuvant erlotinib versus placebo in patients with stage IB-IIIA NSCLC (RADIANT): a randomized, double-blind, Phase III trial. J Clin Oncol 2015. https://doi.org/10.1200/JCO.2015.61.8918.
61. Pennell NA, Neal JW, Chaft JE, et al. SELECT: a phase II trial of adjuvant erlotinib in patients with resected epidermal growth factor receptor-mutant NSCLC. J Clin Oncol 2019;37(2):97–104.
62. Zhong WZ, Wang Q, Mao WM, et al. Gefitinib versus vinorelbine plus cisplatin as adjuvant treatment for stage II–IIIA (N1–N2) EGFR-mutant NSCLC (ADJUVANT/CTONG1104): a randomised, open-label, phase 3 study. Lancet Oncol 2018. https://doi.org/10.1016/S1470-2045(17)30729-5.
63. Yue D, Xu S, Wang Q, et al. Erlotinib versus vinorelbine plus cisplatin as adjuvant therapy in Chinese patients with stage IIIA EGFR mutation-positive NSCLC (EVAN): a randomised, open-label, phase 2 trial. Lancet Respir Med 2018;6(11):863–73.
64. Lu D, Wang Z, Liu X, et al. Differential effects of adjuvant EGFR tyrosine kinase inhibitors in patients with different stages of non-small-cell lung cancer after radical resection: an updated meta-analysis. Cancer Manag Res 2019. https://doi.org/10.2147/CMAR.S187940.
65. Zhong W-Z, Chen K-N, Chen C, et al. Erlotinib versus gemcitabine plus cisplatin as neoadjuvant treatment of stage IIIA-N2 EGFR -mutant non–small-cell lung cancer (EMERGING-CTONG 1103): a randomized phase II study. J Clin Oncol 2019. https://doi.org/10.1200/jco.19.00075.
66. Available at: https://www.amazon.com/AJCC-Cancer-Staging-Manual-Stephen/dp/0387884408/ref=sr_1_fkmr0_1?gclid=EAIaIQobChMI1J6NyPrF5wIVCZyzCh1KUwKSEAAYASAAEgITy_D_BwE&hvadid=345573984463&hvdev=c&hvlocphy=9008341&hvnetw=g&hvpos=1t1&hvqmt=e&hvrand=15196786613092524843&hvtargid=kwd-733802856676&hydadcr=20837_10175449&keywords=ajcc+cancer+staging+manual+8th+ed&qid=1581302433&sr=8-1-fkmr0.

Anaplastic Lymphoma Kinase Mutation–Positive Non–Small Cell Lung Cancer

Anthony V. Serritella, MD[a], Christine M. Bestvina, MD[b,*]

KEYWORDS

• Alectinib • Anaplastic lymphoma kinase (ALK) • Brigatinib • Ceritinib • Crizotinib • Lorlatinib
• Non–small cell lung cancer

KEY POINTS

- Non–small cell lung cancer with anaplastic lymphoma kinase (ALK) chromosomal rearrangement is sensitive to treatment with tyrosine kinase inhibitors (TKIs).
- Numerous TKIs have been developed in recent years, including alectinib, which is the current preferred first-line agent for treatment-naïve patients.
- The development of resistance has led to next-generation ALK inhibitors that better penetrate the central nervous system, which has improved the treatment of brain metastasis.

INTRODUCTION

First described in 2007, echinoderm microtubule-associated protein-like 4 (EML4)-anaplastic lymphoma kinase (ALK) gene rearrangements are chromosomal inversions that lead to constitutive oncogenic activation.[1] Cells harboring ALK rearrangements are sensitive to tyrosine kinase inhibitors (TKIs), which have dramatically improved patient outcomes, with up to 50% of patients surviving 6.8 years after diagnosis.[2]

The proportion of patients with ALK-positive disease varies depending on the population.[3] ALK rearrangements are detected in approximately 3% to 7% of adenocarcinomas,[4] translating to 60,000 new cases annually worldwide.[5] This incidence is similar in Asian (4.2%) and Western (3.4%) populations.[6] ALK-positive disease occurs almost exclusively in adenocarcinomas,[7] is associated with younger age (median age of diagnosis of 52),[8] male sex, and never-smoking or light-smoking history.[3]

ALK-positive patients with stage I–III disease are managed similarly to those with wild-type disease. They may receive surgery, radiation, chemotherapy, or multimodal therapy as appropriate for the patient's stage. It remains to be determined whether TKIs will play a role for these early-stage patients (see later discussion). For patients with previously untreated metastatic ALK-positive disease, multiple TKIs are available (**Table 1**). Drug resistance inevitably emerges, and has led to the development of more potent next-generation ALK inhibitors (**Table 2**).

DIAGNOSTIC TESTING

All patients with metastatic lung adenocarcinoma should be tested for ALK rearrangements[9] using fluorescence in situ hybridization (FISH), immunohistochemistry (IHC), or next-generation sequencing (NGS).[10] FISH is the gold standard for detecting ALK rearrangements, and uses red and green probes to hybridize with either side of

[a] Department of Medicine, University of Chicago Medicine, 5841 South Maryland Avenue, MC 3051, Chicago, IL 60637, USA; [b] Section of Hematology/Oncology, Department of Medicine, University of Chicago Medicine, 5841 South Maryland Avenue, MC2115, Chicago, IL 60637, USA
* Corresponding author.
E-mail address: CBestvina@medicine.bsd.uchicago.edu

Thorac Surg Clin 30 (2020) 137–146
https://doi.org/10.1016/j.thorsurg.2019.12.001

Table 1
Anaplastic lymphoma kinase (ALK) inhibitors as first-line therapy in treatment-naïve ALK-positive patients with non–small cell lung cancer

Drug, Trial Name	Phase	Arms	N	ORR (%)	ORR *P* Value	Median PFS (Months)	PFS *P* Value	OS (Months)	OS *P* Value
Crizotinib, PROFILE 1014[15]	3	Crizotinib	172	74	<.001	10.9	<.001	NR	.0978
		Chemotherapy	171	45		7.0		47.5	
Ceritinib, ASCEND 4[23]	3	Ceritinib	189	72.5	<.01	16.6	<.00001	NR	.056
		Chemotherapy	187	26.7		8.1		26.2	
Alectinib, J-ALEX[34]	3	Alectinib	103	92	NS	34.1[a]	<.0001	NR[a]	NA
		Crizotinib	104	79		10.2[a]		NR[a]	
Alectinib, ALEX[24]	3	Alectinib	152	82.9[b]	.0936	34.8[b]	<.001	NA	NA
		Crizotinib	151	75.5[b]		10.9[b]			
Alectinib, ALESIA[35]	3	Alectinib	125	91	<.01	NR	<.0001	NA	NA
		Crizotinib	62	77		11.1			
Brigatinib, ALTA-1L[38]	3	Brigatinib	137	71	NS	NR[c]	NA	NA	NA
		Crizotinib	138	60		9.8			
Lorlatinib, CROWN[47]	3	Lorlatinib	Ongoing						
		Crizotinib							
Ensartinib, eXALT3[52]	3	Ensartinib	Ongoing						
		Crizotinib							

Abbreviations: NA, not available; NR, not reached; NS, not significant; ORR, objective response rate; OS, overall survival; PFS, progression-free survival.

[a] Follow-up study.[33]

[b] Follow-up study after additional 10 months, Camidge et al.[32]

[c] 12-month PFS rate of 67% with brigatinib versus 43% for crizotinib, *P*<.001.[38]

the ALK translocation breakpoint. These probes either overlay to form a yellow signal for wild-type samples or separate with independent red and green signals if a fusion mutation is present.[11]

An alternative to FISH is IHC, which involves the use of monoclonal antibodies to the ALK fusion oncogene.[12] NGS is performed with extraction of genomic DNA from tumor cells, with probes targeting cancer-specific genes[10] using either plasma or tissue.[13] Comparing these 3 methods, IHC had the greatest positive rate (94.5%), with similar results from NGS (92.7%), followed by FISH (82.4%).[10]

TYROSINE KINASE INHIBITORS

Crizotinib

Crizotinib was the first ALK TKI developed.[14] PROFILE 1007 (N = 347) was a phase 3 trial that compared crizotinib with chemotherapy in patients previously treated with chemotherapy. Crizotinib demonstrated an improvement in objective response rate (ORR) (65% vs 20%, *P*<.001), progression-free survival (PFS) (7.7 months vs 3.0, *P*<.001), and quality of life.[5] In the phase 3 study PROFILE 1014[15] (N = 343), which compared crizotinib with chemotherapy in the front-line setting, crizotinib demonstrated an improved ORR (74% vs 45%, *P*<.001) and PFS (10.9 vs 7.0 months, *P*<.001). In both trials, there was no overall survival (OS) difference, likely because of crossover.[5,16] These trials established the role of crizotinib as the first-line standard of care.

Toxicity

Gastrointestinal toxicity is the most common side effect of crizotinib, including diarrhea (any grade, 61%; grade 3 or 4%, 22%), vomiting (46%), and constipation (43%). Grade 3 or 4 elevated liver function tests (LFTs) was seen in 14% of patients[15]; LFTs should be monitored every 2 weeks for the first 2 months and periodically thereafter. Cardiac toxicity (including bradycardia and QTc prolongation) is also observed. Visual disturbances were seen in 71% of patients, but only 1% were grade 3 or higher.[15]

Central nervous system metastasis

Crizotinib is largely ineffective at controlling central nervous system (CNS) disease, with an intracranial (IC) response rate as low as 7%.[17] The CNS is the most common site of progression for patients on crizotinib.[17] Crizotinib is a known substrate of the drug efflux pump *p*-glycoprotein, limiting its CNS

Table 2
Anaplastic lymphoma kinase (ALK) inhibitors in subsequent-line therapy for previously treated ALK-positive non–small cell lung cancer

Drug, Trial Name	Phase	Prior Therapies	Arms	N	ORR (%)	ORR *P* Value	Median PFS (Months)	PFS *P* Value	OS[a] (Months, HR, or Rate)	OS *P* Value
Crizotinib, PROFILE 1007[5]	3	Platinum-based chemotherapy	Crizotinib Chemotherapy	173 174	65 20	<.001	7.7 3.0	<.001	20.3 mo 22.8 mo	.54
Ceritinib, ASCEND 5[54]	3	Crizotinib, platinum-based chemotherapy	Ceritinib Chemotherapy	115 116	39 7	<.01	5.4 1.6	<.01	1.0[b]	.50
Alectinib, ALUR[36]	3	Chemotherapy Crizotinib	Alectinib Chemotherapy	72 35	37.5 2.9	<.01	7.1 1.6	<.001	NR 12.6 mo	NS
Brigatinib, ALTA[39,43]	2	Crizotinib	Low dose[c] High dose[c]	112 110	48[d] 53[d]	NS	9.2[d] 16.7[d]	NS	29.5 mo[e] 34.1 mo[e]	NA
Lorlatinib, Solomon et al,[46] 2018[f]	2	Crizotinib[g] >1 ALK[g] inhibitor >2 ALK[g] inhibitors	Lorlatinib	59 198 111	70 47 39	NA	NR 7.3 6.9	NA	NA	NA
ASCEND 9[26]	2	Alectinib ± crizotinib	Ceritinib	20	25	NA	3.7	NA	75.6%[h]	NA

Abbreviations: HR, hazard ratio; NA, not available; NS, not significant; ORR, objective response rate; OS, overall survival; PFS, progression-free survival.
[a] OS is reported as either absolute value in months, HR comparing groups, or rate after a specified amount of time.
[b] OS HR reported only.
[c] Low dose represented 90 mg daily, high dose represented 90 mg daily for 7 days followed by 180 mg daily.
[d] Longer-term data released after 8 months of follow-up.[43]
[e] Longer-term data release after greater than 20 months of follow-up.[43]
[f] Selected results only.
[g] Includes those with and without chemotherapy.
[h] 12-month OS rate.

accumulation.[18,19] This lack of CNS efficacy helped drive the development of several next-generation ALK inhibitors.

Ceritinib

Ceritinib is a second-generation ALK inhibitor with activity against IGF-R1, IR, and ROS-1.[20] It has activity in crizotinib-resistant disease, targeting resistance mutations such as the common variants L119M and G1269A, as well as I1171T and S1206Y.[20] Ceritinib also better penetrates the blood-brain barrier.[21]

Ceritinib is approved in both treatment-naïve and crizotinib-resistant patients. ASCEND-5 (N = 231) demonstrated a clinical benefit for ceritinib over third-line chemotherapy in patients previously treated with both platinum-based chemotherapy and crizotinib.[22] ASCEND-4 (N = 376) compared ceritinib with chemotherapy in treatment-naïve patients, including those with asymptomatic or stable brain metastases. Median PFS for the ceritinib group was 16.6 months versus 8.1 months in the chemotherapy group (*P*<.00001).[23] Neither ASCEND-4 nor ASCEND-5 demonstrated an OS benefit, likely because of high crossover. Poor tolerability of ceritinib and the clinical efficacy of alectinib[24] (see later discussion) hindered ceritinib's widespread use.[25]

Whether there will be a role for ceritinib in the treatment of alectinib-resistant disease remains to be seen. ASCEND-9 (N = 20) studied ceritinib in patients who progressed on alectinib and demonstrated an ORR of 25% and disease control rate (DCR) of 70%.[26]

Central nervous system metastasis

Ceritinib has excellent CNS activity with an IC response rate as high as 72%.[27,28] Despite this robust activity, the mean PFS for ceritinib-treated patients with brain metastases was still shorter than those without (10.7 vs 26.3 months).[23] An ongoing phase 2 study ASCEND-7 is evaluating the efficacy and safety of ceritinib in patients with brain metastasis.[29]

Toxicity

Grade 3 or 4 toxicities are seen in as many as 78% of patients.[23] Gastrointestinal toxicity of any grade includes diarrhea (85%), nausea (69%), vomiting (66%), and abdominal pain (25%). More than 70% had grade 3 or worse LFT abnormalities, with notable anorexia and fatigue.[23] Poor tolerability of the approved dose of ceritinib (750 mg once daily while fasting) hindered its adoption,[25] although the new lower dose approved by the Food and Drug Administration (450 mg dose with food) has improved the side effect profile tolerability.[30,31]

Alectinib

Alectinib is a second-generation ALK inhibitor that, owing to robust clinical efficacy and a superior safety profile, is the preferred first-line option for metastatic ALK-positive NSCLC.[9] Alectinib is not a substrate of the *p*-glycoprotein efflux transporter, allowing it to effectively penetrate the CNS.[24]

In the global phase 3 ALEX trial (N = 303), treatment-naïve patients were randomized to first-line alectinib or crizotinib.[24] Median PFS with alectinib was 35 months versus 11 months with crizotinib (hazard ratio [HR] 0.43, *P*<.001),[32,33] although OS data await maturation. Similar results were seen in Japanese patients in J-ALEX (N = 207),[34] as well as a third more recent phase 3 study ALESIA,[35] which compared alectinib with crizotinib in Asian patients. These trials have led to alectinib as the preferred front-line treatment.

In addition, alectinib plays a role in the treatment of patients who progressed on or were intolerant to crizotinib. The phase 3 trial ALUR (N = 107) randomized patients previously treated with chemotherapy and crizotinib to alectinib or chemotherapy. Treatment with alectinib resulted in a PFS of 7.1 months versus 1.6 months in those treated with chemotherapy (HR 0.32, *P*<.01).[36]

Central nervous system metastasis

Excellent CNS activity of alectinib has been consistently demonstrated across all trials. With ALEX, time to CNS progression was significantly longer in the alectinib group compared with the crizotinib group (HR 0.16, *P*<.001).[24] For patients with metastatic CNS disease at baseline, IC responses were achieved in 75% (n = 16) of patients treated with alectinib. Therefore, many patients with CNS disease can be treated with TKIs alone without local therapy (surgery or radiation).

Toxicity

Alectinib is tolerated much better than crizotinib, with grade 3 to 5 toxicities in approximately 40% of patients.[24,34,36] The side-effect profile includes nausea (14%), diarrhea (12%), vomiting (7%),[24] and elevated bilirubin (15%).[24] Alectinib can also cause myalgias (16%),[24] and for this reason creatine kinase (CK) levels are tested every 2 weeks in the first month of therapy. Anemia (20%) and photosensitivity (5%) are also reported.[24]

Brigatinib

Brigatinib is a second-generation oral TKI that can overcome several crizotinib resistance mutations.[37] Brigatinib was granted accelerated approval for treatment of ALK-positive NSCLC in patients who have progressed on crizotinib, with ongoing trials in the front-line setting.

The ALTA-1 trial randomized 275 treatment-naïve patients to brigatinib or crizotinib.[38] PFS at 12 months was improved with brigatinib (67% vs 43%, HR 0.49, *P*<.001). OS in the front-line setting has not yet been released. There are no trials comparing brigatinib with alectinib in the treatment-naïve setting. Brigatinib has showed some promise in crizotinib-refractory patients with PFS as high as 16.7 months in a recent phase 2 trial.[39] There are limited data supporting the use of brigatinib at time of progression on alectinib, with PFS from 4.4 to 6.6 months.[40–42]

Central nervous system metastasis

Brigatinib has excellent IC activity, with 78% (n = 18) of patients with measurable brain metastases at baseline demonstrating an objective IC response (ICR) in the front-line setting.[38] Updated phase 2 results demonstrated that crizotinib-refractory patients with measurable CNS lesions at baseline had a nearly 67% (n = 18 patients) ICR with a median IC PFS of 18.4 months.[43]

Toxicity

In ALTA-1L, grade 3 or higher adverse events occurred in 61% of patients treated with brigatinib (n = 136).[38] Similar to the other ALK inhibitors, the most common adverse events of any grade were gastrointestinal (49%), elevated CK (39%), and increased alanine aminotransferase ALT (19%).[38] Amylase and lipase elevation was also observed (any grade rates of 19% and 14%, respectively), as was cardiac toxicity (particularly bradycardia).[38] Blood pressure should be controlled before brigatinib initiation and monitored monthly,[44] because hypertension has also been observed (n = 136, 23%).[45]

A distinguishing feature of brigatinib is the potential for severe pulmonary toxicity. This typically occurs within 24 to 48 hours of initiation, and manifests as dyspnea and hypoxia with ground-glass opacification and interstitial opacities on imaging.[21] This occurs in 3% to 6% of patients,[21,38,39] appears to be more common in patients with prior crizotinib treatment, and is dose related.[39] Step-up dosing over 7 days is used to mitigate the risk of early pulmonary events.[38,45] For patients with new or worsening respiratory symptoms, brigatinib should be held with prompt evaluation for interstitial lung disease or pneumonitis, and if found to be grade 3 or higher, brigatinib should be discontinued.[44,45]

Lorlatinib

Lorlatinib is a third-generation selective inhibitor of ALK and ROS1.[1] Shaw and colleagues[1] have demonstrated an ORR of 57% (n = 28) for patients harboring the G1202R mutation, commonly found after second-generation ALK inhibitors.

A recent phase 2 study by Solomon and colleagues[46] enrolled 228 ALK-positive patients with a range of prior treatment exposures. Clinical performance varied based on prior TKI exposure. Crizotinib-only patients demonstrated an ORR of 69% (n = 228). Median PFS was not reached. Patients who had failed 2 or more ALK TKIs had a less robust ORR of 39% with PFS of 6.9 months.[46]

An ongoing phase 3 study ("CROWN") is randomizing treatment-naïve ALK-positive NSCLC to either lorlatinib or crizotinib in the first-line setting.[47] A French study, LORLATU (NCT: 02327477) is evaluating treatment sequences in patients receiving lorlatinib.[48] There have not been any studies comparing lorlatinib with chemotherapy in alectinib-resistant disease.

Central nervous system metastasis

The mean cerebrospinal fluid to plasma concentration ratio for lorlatinib was 0.75 in early trials, confirming significant CNS penetration.[49] In patients with baseline brain metastasis previously on at least one ALK inhibitor, lorlatinib had an IC response rate of 63% (n = 81) with median duration of IC response at 14.5 months.

Toxicity

Grade 3 to 4 hyperlipidemia is significant (31%), with 81% of patients requiring a lipid-lowering agent.[50] Peripheral edema of any grade was present in 43% of patients, with peripheral neuropathy in 30%. CNS effects of any grade were reported in 39% of patients including change in cognition (23%), mood (22%), and speech (8%). Most cognitive effects were found to be mild and were rapidly reversible with dose reduction.

TYROSINE KINASE INHIBITORS IN DEVELOPMENT

Ensartinib (X-396) is a novel inhibitor with activity against ALK and ROS1 crizotinib resistance mutations,[51] including L1196M and C1156Y. In a recent phase 1/2 study (N = 60), relative response (RR) rate was 60% with a median PFS of 26.2 months.[51] Activity was seen in patients who had previously received a second-generation ALK TKI (n = 16, ORR 23%, DCR 50%), as well as in patients who had received between 2 and 5 prior regimens of ALK TKIs.[51] Intracranial RR (64%) and IC DCR (92.9%) were particularly promising.[51] A phase 3 trial,[52] eXalt3, is currently comparing ensartinib with crizotinib.

Entrectinib is another novel inhibitor of ALK. A recent phase 1 study found that entrectinib had rapid and durable benefit in patients harboring rearrangements of NTRK, ROS1, and ALK.[53] However, no responses were observed in patients previously treated with ALK inhibitors.[53]

Repotrectinib is a next-generation ROS, TRK-A, and ALK inhibitor that has shown meaningful preliminary clinical activity. The current phase 1/2 trial (Trident-1) is still ongoing.[54]

RESISTANCE MECHANISMS

Mutations in the ALK kinase domain are the best described mechanism of TKI resistance,[55] occurring in both crizotinib-treated patients (20%–36%)[56,57] and patients treated with a second-generation ALK inhibitor (>50%). Each TKI is associated with an individual spectrum of mutations.[14,57] Gainor and colleagues[57] analyzed 103 biopsies from ALK-positive patients progressing on various ALK inhibitors. L1196M is the most common mutation found in crizotinib resistance (7%).[57] G1202R occurs frequently after second-generation agents, including ceritinib (21%), alectinib (29%), and brigatinib (43%).[16,36,45,58] Even though G1202R confers high-level resistance, it can be overcome by lorlatinib.[57,58] Little is known regarding lorlatinib resistance.

Resistance mechanisms outside of the ALK kinase domain also occur. Amplification of the ALK domain occurs in about 10% of crizotinib-resistant samples, either in isolation or with other mutations.[59,60] Bypass signaling pathway activation is another resistance mechanism, with activation of the epidermal growth factor receptor (EGFR) most commonly reported.[59,61] Transformation to both spindle-cell morphology[62] and squamous cell lung cancer have also been described.[58,63]

SYSTEMIC THERAPY AFTER TYROSINE KINASE INHIBITORS

Treatment with chemotherapy, with or without immunotherapy, is used after targeted therapies have been exhausted. The use of combination chemoimmunotherapy is supported by a subgroup analysis of 111 patients with EGFR and ALK mutations from the IMpower150 study.[64] The combination of carboplatin, paclitaxel, bevacizumab, and atezolizumab demonstrated an improvement of PFS in patients with EGFR and ALK mutations over carboplatin, paclitaxel, and bevacizumab (9.7 months vs 6.1 months; HR 0.59, 95% confidence interval 0.37–0.94).

Outside of IMpower150, data supporting the use of immunotherapy in ALK-mutated patients is scarce. Patients with ALK mutations were excluded from KEYNOTE-189, which studied the combination of carboplatin, pemetrexed, and pembrolizumab.[65] Negative clinical trial results were seen for ALK patients with carboplatin/nab-paclitaxel/atezolizumab,[66,67] nivolumab,[68] pembrolizumab,[69] and atezolizumab.[70] In addition, extrapolation of EGFR data lead to safety concerns in giving TKI therapy either with[71] or following immunotherapy.[72] Testing for ALK should be completed before the administration of chemoimmunotherapy in the untreated setting to avoid this increased toxicity risk.

DISCUSSION

Alectinib is the current preferred first-line treatment for ALK-positive, metastatic NSCLC.[9] This preference is based on improved efficacy, side-effect profile, and CNS activity when compared with crizotinib.[24,34] Brigatinib, ceritinib, and crizotinib remain options for front-line treatment, and may be considered based on individual clinical circumstances. Lorlatinib should be considered after progression on alectinib.

Excellent CNS activity of alectinib and brigatinib has allowed for treatment of CNS metastasis with TKI therapy and has allowed patients to delay or avoid the use of radiotherapy or surgery for local control.[24,27,28,39,43] For patients with CNS progression on alectinib, lorlatinib remains an option.[49]

FUTURE DIRECTIONS

Long-term follow-up data for brigatinib await maturity, and how this drug will compare with alectinib remains to be seen. Ensartinib, entrectinib, and repotrectinib are all being investigated in clinical trials, and the role they will play is yet to be determined. Additional data are needed regarding the optimal treatment following TKI therapy, whether it be chemotherapy or chemoimmunotherapy.

The role of TKIs in the perioperative setting is under investigation. Crizotinib is being studied in the neoadjuvant setting[73] as well as the adjuvant setting as part of the larger, multi-institutional Adjuvant Lung Cancer Enrichment Marker Identification and Sequencing Trial (ALCHEMIST).[74,75] An ongoing phase 3 study (ALINA) is evaluating the efficacy and safety of alectinib compared with platinum-based chemotherapy in patients with completed resected IB to stage IIIA tumors as an adjuvant therapy.[76]

In summary, excellent progress has been made over the past decade in the treatment of ALK-positive NSCLC, with 4 TKIs now approved in the front-line setting, with additional options available at time of progression. Next-generation ALK inhibitors demonstrate excellent CNS response rates. Future areas of research include additional next-generation TKIs, the perioperative role of TKIs, and the optimal systemic treatment once TKI options have been exhausted.

DISCLOSURE

Dr A.V. Serritella has nothing to disclose. Dr C.M. Bestvina discloses the following: Consulting: AbbVie, AstraZeneca, Genentech, Pfizer. Honorarium: OncLive. Travel: EMD Serono.

REFERENCES

1. Shaw AT, Solomon BJ, Besse B, et al. ALK resistance mutations and efficacy of lorlatinib in advanced anaplastic lymphoma kinase-positive non-small-cell lung cancer. J Clin Oncol 2019; 37(16):1370–9.
2. Pacheco JM, Gao D, Smith D, et al. Natural history and factors associated with overall survival in stage IV ALK-rearranged non-small cell lung cancer. J Thorac Oncol 2019;14(4):691–700.
3. Hofman P. ALK in Non-Small Cell Lung Cancer (NSCLC) pathobiology, epidemiology, detection from tumor tissue and algorithm diagnosis in a daily practice. Cancers (Basel) 2017;9(8):107.
4. Pikor LA, Ramnarine VR, Lam S, et al. Genetic alterations defining NSCLC subtypes and their therapeutic implications. Lung Cancer 2013;82(2):179–89.
5. Shaw AT, Kim DW, Nakagawa K, et al. Crizotinib versus chemotherapy in advanced ALK-positive lung cancer. N Engl J Med 2013;368(25):2385–94.
6. Solomon B, Varella-Garcia M, Camidge DR. ALK gene rearrangements: a new therapeutic target in a molecularly defined subset of non-small cell lung cancer. J Thorac Oncol 2009;4(12):1450–4.
7. Boland JM, Erdogan S, Vasmatzis G, et al. Anaplastic lymphoma kinase immunoreactivity correlates with ALK gene rearrangement and transcriptional up-regulation in non-small cell lung carcinomas. Hum Pathol 2009;40(8):1152–8.
8. Shaw AT, Yeap BY, Mino-Kenudson M, et al. Clinical features and outcome of patients with non-small-cell lung cancer who harbor EML4-ALK. J Clin Oncol 2009;27(26):4247–53.
9. National Comprehensive Cancer N. Non small cell lung cancer (Version 6.2019). Available at: http://www.nccn.org/professionals/physician_gls/f_guidelines.asp. Accessed August 23, 2019.
10. Lin C, Shi X, Yang S, et al. Comparison of ALK detection by FISH, IHC and NGS to predict benefit from crizotinib in advanced non-small-cell lung cancer. Lung Cancer 2019;131:62–8.
11. Martelli MP, Sozzi G, Hernandez L, et al. EML4-ALK rearrangement in non-small cell lung cancer and non-tumor lung tissues. Am J Pathol 2009;174(2):661–70.
12. Conklin CM, Craddock KJ, Have C, et al. Immunohistochemistry is a reliable screening tool for identification of ALK rearrangement in non-small-cell lung carcinoma and is antibody dependent. J Thorac Oncol 2013;8(1):45–51.
13. Supplee JG, Milan MSD, Lim LP, et al. Sensitivity of next-generation sequencing assays detecting oncogenic fusions in plasma cell-free DNA. Lung Cancer 2019;134:96–9.
14. Awad MM, Shaw AT. ALK inhibitors in non-small cell lung cancer: crizotinib and beyond. Clin Adv Hematol Oncol 2014;12(7):429–39.
15. Solomon BJ, Mok T, Kim DW, et al. First-line crizotinib versus chemotherapy in ALK-positive lung cancer. N Engl J Med 2014;371(23):2167–77.
16. Solomon BJ, Kim D-W, Wu Y-L, et al. Final overall survival analysis from a study comparing first-line crizotinib versus chemotherapy in ALK-mutation-positive non-small-cell lung cancer. J Clin Oncol 2018;36(22):2251–8.
17. Costa DB, Shaw AT, Ou SH, et al. Clinical experience with crizotinib in patients with advanced ALK-rearranged non-small-cell lung cancer and brain metastases. J Clin Oncol 2015;33(17):1881–8.
18. Metro G, Lunardi G, Floridi P, et al. CSF concentration of crizotinib in two ALK-positive non-small-cell lung cancer patients with CNS metastases deriving clinical benefit from treatment. J Thorac Oncol 2015;10(5):e26–7.
19. Tang SC, Nguyen LN, Sparidans RW, et al. Increased oral availability and brain accumulation of the ALK inhibitor crizotinib by coadministration of the P-glycoprotein (ABCB1) and breast cancer resistance protein (ABCG2) inhibitor elacridar. Int J Cancer 2014;134(6):1484–94.
20. Friboulet L, Li N, Katayama R, et al. The ALK inhibitor ceritinib overcomes crizotinib resistance in non-small cell lung cancer. Cancer Discov 2014; 4(6):662–73.
21. Dagogo-Jack I, Shaw AT, Riely GJ. Optimizing treatment for patients with anaplastic lymphoma kinase-positive lung cancer. Clin Pharmacol Ther 2017; 101(5):625–33.
22. Shaw AT, Kim TM, Crino L, et al. Ceritinib versus chemotherapy in patients with ALK-rearranged non-small-cell lung cancer previously given chemotherapy and crizotinib (ASCEND-5): a randomised, controlled, open-label, phase 3 trial. Lancet Oncol 2017;18(7):874–86.
23. Soria JC, Tan DSW, Chiari R, et al. First-line ceritinib versus platinum-based chemotherapy in advanced ALK-rearranged non-small-cell lung cancer (ASCEND-4): a randomised, open-label, phase 3 study. Lancet 2017;389(10072):917–29.
24. Peters S, Camidge DR, Shaw AT, et al. Alectinib versus crizotinib in untreated ALK-positive non-small-cell lung cancer. N Engl J Med 2017;377(9):829–38.

25. Wu F, Ou S-HI. ASCEND-5: too little too late? J Thorac Dis 2017;9(10):3477–9.
26. Hida T, Seto T, Horinouchi H, et al. Phase II study of ceritinib in alectinib-pretreated patients with anaplastic lymphoma kinase-rearranged metastatic non-small-cell lung cancer in Japan: ASCEND-9. Cancer Sci 2018;109(9):2863–72.
27. Crino L, Ahn MJ, De Marinis F, et al. Multicenter phase II study of whole-body and intracranial activity with ceritinib in patients with ALK-rearranged non-small-cell lung cancer previously treated with chemotherapy and crizotinib: results from ASCEND-2. J Clin Oncol 2016;34(24):2866–73.
28. Kim DW, Mehra R, Tan DSW, et al. Activity and safety of ceritinib in patients with ALK-rearranged non-small-cell lung cancer (ASCEND-1): updated results from the multicentre, open-label, phase 1 trial. Lancet Oncol 2016;17(4):452–63.
29. LDK378 versus chemotherapy in ALK rearranged (ALK Positive) patients previously treated with chemotherapy (Platinum Doublet) and Crizotinib. Available at: https://clinicaltrials.gov/ct2/show/NCT01828112. Accessed August 23, 2019.
30. Cho BC, Kim DW, Bearz A, et al. ASCEND-8: a randomized phase 1 study of ceritinib, 450 mg or 600 mg, taken with a low-fat meal versus 750 mg in fasted state in patients with anaplastic lymphoma kinase (ALK)-rearranged metastatic non-small cell lung cancer (NSCLC). J Thorac Oncol 2017;12(9):1357–67.
31. Certinib capsules. United States prescribing information. US National Library of Medicine. Available at: http://accessdata.fda.gov/drugsatfda_docs/label/2017/205755s009lbl.pdf. Accessed August 23, 2019.
32. Camidge DR, Dziadziuszko R, Peters S, et al. Updated efficacy and safety data and impact of the EML4-ALK fusion variant on the efficacy of alectinib in untreated ALK-positive advanced non-small cell lung cancer in the global phase III ALEX study. J Thorac Oncol 2019;14(7):1233–43.
33. Seto T, Nishio M, Hida T, et al. Final PFS analysis and safety data from the phase III J-ALEX study of alectinib (ALC) vs. crizotinib (CRZ) in ALK-inhibitor naïve ALK-positive non-small cell lung cancer (ALK+ NSCLC). J Clin Oncol 2019;37(15_suppl):9092.
34. Hida T, Nokihara H, Kondo M, et al. Alectinib versus crizotinib in patients with ALK-positive non-small-cell lung cancer (J-ALEX): an open-label, randomised phase 3 trial. Lancet 2017;390(10089):29–39.
35. Zhou C, Kim SW, Reungwetwattana T, et al. Alectinib versus crizotinib in untreated Asian patients with anaplastic lymphoma kinase-positive non-small-cell lung cancer (ALESIA): a randomised phase 3 study. Lancet Respir Med 2019;7(5):437–46.
36. Novello S, Mazieres J, Oh IJ, et al. Alectinib versus chemotherapy in crizotinib-pretreated anaplastic lymphoma kinase (ALK)-positive non-small-cell lung cancer: results from the phase III ALUR study. Ann Oncol 2018;29(6):1409–16.
37. Zhang S, Anjum R, Squillace R, et al. The potent ALK inhibitor brigatinib (AP26113) overcomes mechanisms of resistance to first- and second-generation ALK inhibitors in preclinical models. Clin Cancer Res 2016;22(22):5527–38.
38. Camidge DR, Kim HR, Ahn M-J, et al. Brigatinib versus crizotinib in ALK-positive non–small-cell lung cancer. N Engl J Med 2018;379(21):2027–39.
39. Kim DW, Tiseo M, Ahn MJ, et al. Brigatinib in patients with crizotinib-refractory anaplastic lymphoma kinase-positive non-small-cell lung cancer: a randomized, multicenter phase II trial. J Clin Oncol 2017;35(22):2490–8.
40. Descourt R, Perol M, Rousseau-Bussac G, et al. Brigatinib in pretreated patients with ALK-positive advanced NSCLC. J Clin Oncol 2019;37(15_suppl):9045.
41. Lin JJ, Zhu VW, Schoenfeld AJ, et al. Brigatinib in patients with alectinib-refractory ALK-positive NSCLC. J Thorac Oncol 2018;13(10):1530–8.
42. Stinchcombe T, Doebele RC, Wang XF, et al. Preliminary results of single arm phase 2 trial of brigatinib in patients (pts) with progression disease (PD) after next-generation (NG) anaplastic lymphoma kinase (ALK) tyrosine kinase inhibitors (TKIs) in ALK + non-small cell lung cancer (NSCLC). J Clin Oncol 2019;37(15_suppl):9027.
43. Huber RM, Kim D-W, Ahn M-J, et al. Brigatinib (BRG) in crizotinib (CRZ)-refractory ALK+ non–small cell lung cancer (NSCLC): efficacy updates and exploratory analysis of CNS ORR and overall ORR by baseline (BL) brain lesion status. J Clin Oncol 2018;36(15_suppl):9061.
44. Brigatinib capsules. United States prescribing information. US National Library of Medicine. Available at: https://www.accessdata.fda.gov/drugsatfda_docs/label/2017/208772lbl.pdf. Accessed August 23, 2019.
45. Camidge DR, Pabani A, Miller RM, et al. Management strategies for early-onset pulmonary events associated with brigatinib. J Thorac Oncol 2019;14(9):1547–55.
46. Solomon BJ, Besse B, Bauer TM, et al. Lorlatinib in patients with ALK-positive non-small-cell lung cancer: results from a global phase 2 study. Lancet Oncol 2018;19(12):1654–67.
47. A Study of lorlatinib versus crizotinib in first line treatment of patients with ALK-positive NSCLC. Available at: https://ClinicalTrials.gov/show/NCT03052608. Accessed August 23, 2019.
48. Efficacy of treatment sequences in patients with non-small cell lung cancer receiving Lorlatinib. Available at: https://ClinicalTrials.gov/show/NCT03727477. Accessed August 23, 2019.

49. Shaw AT, Felip E, Bauer TM, et al. Lorlatinib in non-small-cell lung cancer with ALK or ROS1 rearrangement: an international, multicentre, open-label, single-arm first-in-man phase 1 trial. Lancet Oncol 2017;18(12):1590–9.
50. Bauer TM, Felip E, Solomon BJ, et al. Clinical management of adverse events associated with Lorlatinib. Oncologist 2019;24(8):1103–10.
51. Horn L, Infante JR, Reckamp KL, et al. Ensartinib (X-396) in ALK-positive non-small cell lung cancer: results from a first-in-human phase I/II, multicenter study. Clin Cancer Res 2018;24(12):2771–9.
52. eXalt3: study comparing X-396 (ensartinib) to crizotinib in ALK positive non-small cell lung cancer (NSCLC) patients. Available at: https://ClinicalTrials.gov/show/NCT02767804. Accessed August 23, 2019.
53. Drilon A, Siena S, Ou SI, et al. Safety and antitumor activity of the multitargeted Pan-TRK, ROS1, and ALK inhibitor entrectinib: combined results from two phase I trials (ALKA-372-001 and STARTRK-1). Cancer Discov 2017;7(4):400–9.
54. A study of repotrectinib (TPX-0005) in patients with advanced solid tumors harboring ALK, ROS1, or NTRK1-3 rearrangements. Available at: https://ClinicalTrials.gov/show/NCT03093116. Accessed August 23, 2019.
55. Choi YL, Soda M, Yamashita Y, et al. EML4-ALK mutations in lung cancer that confer resistance to ALK inhibitors. N Engl J Med 2010;363(18):1734–9.
56. Doebele RC, Pilling AB, Aisner DL, et al. Mechanisms of resistance to crizotinib in patients with ALK gene rearranged non-small cell lung cancer. Clin Cancer Res 2012;18(5):1472–82.
57. Gainor JF, Dardaei L, Yoda S, et al. Molecular mechanisms of resistance to first- and second-generation ALK inhibitors in ALK-rearranged lung cancer. Cancer Discov 2016;6(10):1118–33.
58. Qiao H, Lovly CM. Cracking the code of resistance across multiple lines of ALK inhibitor therapy in lung cancer. Cancer Discov 2016;6(10):1084–6.
59. Katayama R, Shaw AT, Khan TM, et al. Mechanisms of acquired crizotinib resistance in ALK-rearranged lung Cancers. Sci Transl Med 2012;4(120):120ra117.
60. Salido M, Pijuan L, Martinez-Aviles L, et al. Increased ALK gene copy number and amplification are frequent in non-small cell lung cancer. J Thorac Oncol 2011;6(1):21–7.
61. Sasaki T, Okuda K, Zheng W, et al. The neuroblastoma-associated F1174L ALK mutation causes resistance to an ALK kinase inhibitor in ALK-translocated cancers. Cancer Res 2010;70(24):10038–43.
62. Fukuda K, Takeuchi S, Arai S, et al. Epithelial-to-mesenchymal transition is a mechanism of ALK inhibitor resistance in lung cancer independent of ALK mutation status. Cancer Res 2019;79(7):1658–70.
63. Takigawa N. How should we treat alectinib-refractory ALK-positive non-small cell lung cancer? J Thorac Oncol 2018;13(10):1438–40.
64. Socinski MA, Jotte RM, Cappuzzo F, et al. Atezolizumab for first-line treatment of metastatic nonsquamous NSCLC. N Engl J Med 2018;378(24):2288–301.
65. Gandhi L, Rodríguez-Abreu D, Gadgeel S, et al. Pembrolizumab plus chemotherapy in metastatic non–small-cell lung cancer. N Engl J Med 2018;378(22):2078–92.
66. Cappuzzo F, McCleod M, Hussein M, et al. LBA53IMpower130: Progression-free survival (PFS) and safety analysis from a randomised phase III study of carboplatin + nab-paclitaxel (CnP) with or without atezolizumab (atezo) as first-line (1L) therapy in advanced non-squamous NSCLC. Ann Oncol 2018;29(suppl_8). https://doi.org/10.1093/annonc/mdy424.065.
67. Reck M, Mok TSK, Nishio M, et al. Atezolizumab plus bevacizumab and chemotherapy in non-small-cell lung cancer (IMpower150): key subgroup analyses of patients with EGFR mutations or baseline liver metastases in a randomised, open-label phase 3 trial. Lancet Respir Med 2019;7(5):387–401.
68. Borghaei H, Paz-Ares L, Horn L, et al. Nivolumab versus docetaxel in advanced nonsquamous non-small-cell lung cancer. N Engl J Med 2015;373(17):1627–39.
69. Herbst RS, Baas P, Kim DW, et al. Pembrolizumab versus docetaxel for previously treated, PD-L1-positive, advanced non-small-cell lung cancer (KEYNOTE-010): a randomised controlled trial. Lancet 2016;387(10027):1540–50.
70. Rittmeyer A, Barlesi F, Waterkamp D, et al. Atezolizumab versus docetaxel in patients with previously treated non-small-cell lung cancer (OAK): a phase 3, open-label, multicentre randomised controlled trial. Lancet 2017;389(10066):255–65.
71. Chih-Hsin Yang J, Shepherd FA, Kim DW, et al. Osimertinib plus durvalumab versus osimertinib monotherapy in EGFR T790M-positive NSCLC following previous EGFR TKI therapy: CAURAL brief report. J Thorac Oncol 2019;14(5):933–9.
72. Schoenfeld AJ, Arbour KC, Rizvi H, et al. Severe immune-related adverse events are common with sequential PD-(L)1 blockade and osimertinib. Ann Oncol 2019;30(5):839–44.
73. Evaluating crizotinib in the neoadjuvant setting in patients with non-small cell lung cancer. Available at: https://ClinicalTrials.gov/show/NCT03088930. Accessed August 23, 2019.

74. Genetic testing in screening patients with stage IB-IIIA non-small cell lung cancer that has been or will be removed by surgery (The ALCHEMIST Screening Trial). Available at: https://ClinicalTrials.gov/show/NCT02194738. Accessed August 23, 2019.
75. Crizotinib in treating patients with stage IB-IIIA non-small cell lung cancer that has been removed by surgery and ALK fusion mutations (An ALCHEMIST Treatment Trial). Available at: https://clinicaltrials.gov/ct2/show/NCT02201992. Accessed July 30, 2019.
76. Solomon BJ, Ahn JS, Barlesi F, et al. ALINA: a phase III study of alectinib versus chemotherapy as adjuvant therapy in patients with stage IB-IIIA anaplastic lymphoma kinase-positive (ALK+) non-small cell lung cancer (NSCLC). J Clin Oncol 2019;37(15_suppl):TPS8569.

ROS1-rearranged Non–small Cell Lung Cancer

Nicholas P. Giustini, MD[a], Lyudmila Bazhenova, MD[b,*]

KEYWORDS

• Lung cancer • Non–small cell lung cancer (NSCLC) • ROS1 fusion • ROS1 rearrangement • ROS1 inhibitor • Tyrosine kinase inhibitor (TKI) • Targeted therapy • Resistance mechanism

KEY POINTS

- ROS1-rearranged non–small cell lung cancer (NSCLC) makes up 1% to 2% of all NSCLC.
- The ROS1 kinase is fused with a partner leading to constitutive activation of the ROS1 kinase domain with subsequent phosphorylation and activation of downstream signaling.
- Identification of ROS1 is done through immunohistochemistry, fluorescence in situ hybridization, reverse transcription polymerase chain reaction, and next-generation sequencing.
- Treatment includes the use of TKIs targeting the activated ROS1 kinase, including first-line use of crizotinib and entrectinib.
- The main secondary resistance mutations include L2026M, G2032R, G2033N, and S1986Y/F.

INTRODUCTION

According to the World Health Organization in 2018, lung cancer is tied with breast cancer for highest yearly incidence of cancer and is by far the largest cause of cancer-related mortality. Non–small cell lung cancer (NSCLC) comprises approximately 85% of all lung cancers, with genetic alterations in epidermal growth factor receptor (EGFR) entailing 10% to 25% of NSCLC and anaplastic lymphoma kinase (ALK) fusions making up another 5%, with higher relative percentages among both in nonsmokers. In patients with metastatic disease and an oncogenic driver (the sole genetic alteration leading to malignant proliferation), the use of oral medications to block this driver has been shown to be effective in managing this malignancy.[1] ROS1 rearrangements are estimated to occur in 1% to 2% of NSCLCs and are amenable to tyrosine kinase inhibitor (TKI) therapy.[2]

ROS1 MOLECULAR BASIS

In the 1980s, ROS1 was discovered as the oncogenic product of the chicken UR2 sarcoma virus and subsequently identified as proto-oncogenic in human glioblastoma cells.[3–5] ROS1 is related to ALK, LTK, and the insulin receptor families, and the unaltered gene encodes a receptor tyrosine kinase, although a physiologic ligand has yet to be identified. ROS1 rearrangements have been reported in glioblastoma, NSCLC, cholangiocarcinoma, ovarian carcinoma, angiosarcoma, inflammatory myofibroblastic tumors, and spitzoid melanocytic tumors, among others.[6]

The initial ROS1 fusion partner identified was FIG (found in glioblastoma) and is generated by an intrachromosomal homozygous deletion on 6q21 leading to the amino terminal of FIG attaching to and constitutively activating the carboxy terminal kinase of ROS1.[7] Numerous other ROS1 fusion partners exist in NSCLC, including but not limited to CD74, EZR, SDC4, TPM3, GOPC, ZCCHC8, SCL34A2, CCDC6, MYO5C, GPRC6A, LRIG3, CTNND2, OPRM1, and SRSF6.[6,8] In vitro studies have shown that constitutive autophosphorylation of ROS1 leads to phosphorylation of SHP-2 and in turn phosphorylation of MAP/ERK kinase, ERK, STAT3, and AKT. In contrast, phosphorylation of these signals has been shown to

[a] UCSD Moores Cancer Center, 3855 Health Sciences Drive #0829, La Jolla, CA 92093-0829, USA; [b] UCSD Moores Cancer Center, 3855 Health Sciences Drive MC #0987, La Jolla, CA 92093-0829, USA
* Corresponding author.
E-mail address: lbazhenova@health.ucsd.edu

Thorac Surg Clin 30 (2020) 147–156
https://doi.org/10.1016/j.thorsurg.2020.01.007

thoracic.theclinics.com

be decreased in the presence of ROS1 inhibitors.[9–11]

ROS1 and ALK share approximately 49% homology within the kinase domain, and possibly even higher homology within the ATP-binding pocket, indicating likely cross-activity between originally designed ALK inhibitors and ROS1 targets.[12] In vitro crizotinib binds more tightly and seems to be 5 times more potent against ROS1 than ALK fusion cell lines, likely indicating higher inhibition of ROS1 fusions at studied crizotinib doses.[13]

Testing

Fluorescence in situ hybridization

Fluorescence in situ hybridization (FISH) is a technique that can identify the ROS1 fusion partner and is often considered the definitive standard. FISH involves labeling the 3' (centromeric) portion of the fusion breakpoint with a fluorochrome and the 5' (telomeric) portion with a different-colored fluorochrome in order to identify when they have been split apart. There are 2 possible positive rearrangement patterns:

- Classic (break-apart) pattern: 1 normal fusion signal (native ROS1) with 2 separated 3′ and 5′ signals
- Atypical (isolated 3′ signal) pattern: 1 normal fusion signal (native ROS1) with 1 3′ signal without the corresponding 5′ signal

Thresholds for FISH positivity usually involve the presence of greater than 15% split signals (including both classic and atypical patterns).[14,15]

Immunohistochemistry

Immunohistochemistry (IHC) uses the D4D6 monoclonal rabbit antibody to stain slides for ROS1 protein positivity. The scoring for IHC positivity ranges from 0 to 3+ with slight variations in the definitions between different categories. Broadly, they are:

- 0 = No detectable staining in tumor cells
- 1+ = Faint cytoplasmic staining in tumor cells that does not exceed background cell staining
- 2+ = Cytoplasmic staining exceeding background cell staining in 0% to 50% of tumor cells
- 3+ = Cytoplasmic staining exceeding background cell staining in greater than 50% of tumor cells

IHC staining is inexpensive and fast; however, the International Association for the Study of Lung Cancer (IASLC) recommends that although it may be used as a screening tool, there should be confirmation of ROS1 positivity via a complementary method.[15,16]

Multiple studies have shown the potential use of IHC as a screening tool given its high relative sensitivity to specificity, depending on the IHC staining cutoff chosen compared with FISH. For instance, 1 study showed a cutoff of 2+ or higher provided a sensitivity of 100% and specificity of 92%, whereas a cutoff of 3+ only provided a sensitivity of 87.5% and specificity of 98%.[17] Similarly, a separate study showed a sensitivity of 100% and specificity of 97.8% with an IHC cutoff of 2+ or greater.[15] Although most studies indicate sensitivity close to 100% with an IHC cutoff of 2+ or higher, 1 study did note a sensitivity of 76.9% and specificity of 95.7% with an IHC of 2+ or higher compared with a sensitivity of 100% and specificity of 93.6% with an IHC of 1+ or higher.[18–20]

False-positivity of IHC can be related to numerous factors. For instance, in 1 study, most invasive mucinous adenocarcinomas showed ROS1 reactivity on IHC with no ROS1 fusion found, possibly related to artifact from mucin. In addition, nonmalignant areas of biopsy samples can stain positive on IHC, including in osteoclast-type giant cells and in areas of type II pneumocyte hyperplasia and bronchiolar metaplasia.[17,18,21]

Reverse transcriptase polymerase chain reaction

Reverse transcriptase (RT) polymerase chain reaction (PCR) testing uses RNA reverse transcribed into complementary DNA, and then amplified using specific ROS1 gene fusion primers via PCR, and subsequently sequenced for confirmation. The main drawbacks of RT-PCR include the requirement for a larger amount of tissue, inability to identify fusions that are not prespecified, and a higher false-positive rate. One study noted that although 100% of FISH-positive samples were identified by RT-PCR, only 65% of RT-PCR–positive samples are FISH positive with a sensitivity of 100% and a specificity of 85.1%. False-positives are posited to be from small subsets of tumor cells with ROS1 positivity, detected by the amplification of PCR, or RNA that is present on the transcriptional level that does not undergo further translation and is likely not clinically significant.[14,15,20,22]

Next-generation sequencing

Next-generation sequencing uses sequencing in parallel on a massive scale to identify a large number of separate genetic alterations. Individual DNA or RNA is separated spatially and undergoes amplification to eventually identify predetermined genes. Amplification can be achieved either through the use of amplicon sequencing via multiple PCR reactions or hybrid capture sequencing. Sequencing in parallel of the predetermined genes in combination with computational data processing allows the organization and identification of genetic alterations, including gene rearrangements.[16] An RNA-based anchored multiplex PCR assay of 319 fixed paraffin-embedded samples showed a 100% sensitivity and 100% specificity of gene rearrangement identification compared with FISH.[22]

ROS1 CLINICAL DATA

Crizotinib

Given ALK and ROS kinase domain homology, success with crizotinib in ALK fusion–positive NSCLC, and evidence of more effective binding of crizotinib at tolerated doses, crizotinib became the first TKI to be investigated to target ROS1 fusion–positive NSCLC at the dose of 250 mg by mouth twice a day. An early retrospective analysis evaluated the efficacy of different therapies in a ROS1 fusion–positive NSCLC population of 51 patients. The 15 patients who received crizotinib in the second line or later were compared with 49 patients who received pemetrexed-based chemotherapy in any line of therapy versus 44 patients who received non–pemetrexed-based chemotherapy in any line of therapy. Progression-free survival (PFS) was 294 days in the crizotinib group versus 179 days in the pemetrexed-based chemotherapy group and 110 days in the non–pemetrexed-based chemotherapy group. When evaluating the pemetrexed-based chemotherapy group, when patients are split into those with tumors that express low levels of thymidylate synthetase (TS) messenger RNA (mRNA) versus high levels, the PFS further separates to 184 days versus 110 days.[23]

These data show a similar hypothesis as in ALK NSCLC, that patients with ALK or ROS1 fusions may be more susceptible to pemetrexed-based chemotherapy because of decreased TS levels as a result of the driver mutation.[24] Some controversy exists, because a separate retrospective analysis evaluating the use of pemetrexed-based chemotherapy in patients with different driver mutations found a PFS of 7.5 months in ROS1 patients, 5.3 months in with ALK fusion, 3.7 months in EGFR-mutated patients, and 4.1 months in nondriver patients, which was statistically significant, although the sample size of ROS1 patients was small. In this group of patients, although patients with ROS1 fusion seemed to respond to pemetrexed-based therapy for longer, there was no correlation with TS levels.[25]

The first prospective evaluation of crizotinib in ROS1 fusion-positive NSCLC was in PROFILE 1001, an expansion cohort of the phase I study of crizotinib as a MET and ALK inhibitor, which found the maximum tolerable dose of crizotinib to be 250 mg by mouth twice a day.[26] Fifty patients with advanced NSCLC with ROS1 rearrangements, largely previously treated, received crizotinib and showed an overall response rate (ORR) of 72% and a disease control rate (DCR) of 90%. Median PFS was 19.2 months and the overall survival (OS) rate at 12 months was 85%. PFS results of crizotinib in ROS1-rearranged NSCLC were promising and more than doubled that of ALK-rearranged NSCLC (PFS of 9.1 months).[27] Recently updated results of PROFILE 1001 were published showing a median PFS of 19.3 months and a median OS of 51.4 months.[28]

Soon after the publication of PROFILE 1001, multiple other studies reported the efficacy of crizotinib with ROS1-rearranged NSCLC. In the EUROS1 retrospective analysis of 31 patients with previously treated ROS1-rearranged NSCLC, the ORR was 80% and DCR was 86.6%, similar to PROFILE 1001. However, median PFS was noted as much lower, at 9.1 months.[29] A much larger phase II study in East Asia was conducted with 127 largely previously treated patients with ROS1-rearranged NSCLC showing an ORR of 71.7% and DCR of 88.2%. Median PFS was 15.9 months and a 12-month OS was 83.1%. Interestingly, when separating patients into those with baseline brain metastases and those without, median PFS was 10.2 months and 18.8 months, respectively.[30] These data may elucidate the higher PFS in PROFILE 1001 given originally patients with brain metastases were excluded and only later allowed by amendment, likely indicating enrollment of fewer of these patients.[27]

Three trials (EUCROSS, AcSé, and METROS) are ongoing to evaluate the efficacy of crizotinib in ROS1-rearranged NSCLC. In the EUCROSS trial, the 18 patients treated showed an ORR of 83%. In the AcSé trial, the 37 patients treated showed an ORR of 71%, a DCR of 85%, and a median PFS of 10 months. The METROS trial has no reportable data.[31,32]

An additional retrospective analysis of 49 patients with ROS1-rearranged NSCLC was completed in 2018, which showed an ORR of 83.3% and DCR of 97.2%. Median PFS was 12.6 months and median OS was 32.7 months. A further analysis was completed to evaluate for differences in outcomes when stratified for ROS1 fusion partners, with CD74 as the most common fusion partner (52.8% of patients analyzed). Differences in PFS between CD74 fusions and non-

CD74 fusions were 12.6 months and 17.6 months respectively. Differences in OS between CD74 fusions and non-CD74 fusions were 24.3 months and 44.5 months. Both PFS and OS differences trended toward significance; however, on multivariate analysis, they were not found to be statistically significant. A confounding factor for worse prognosis may have been brain metastases, given that only patients with CD74 fusions at initiation of crizotinib had brain disease, with no patients with non-CD74 fusion found to have brain metastases; brain metastases before crizotinib treatment was an independent poor prognostic factor. However, although these data may indicate that brain metastases are more common in patients with CD74-ROS1 NSCLC, during treatment an equivalent percentage of CD74 and non-CD74 patients developed brain metastases. The small sample sizes limit the ability to generalize; however, it does raise the question of whether or not patients with CD74-ROS1 NSCLC develop brain metastases earlier than other fusions and subsequently do worse.[33]

A separate analysis of ROS1 fusion partners was completed on the 127-patient East Asian cohort discussed earlier. Again, CD74 was the most common fusion partner for ROS1, with 49.1% of samples analyzed containing this fusion. When comparing different pairs, including CD74, SDC4, non-CD74, and non-SDC4 in different combinations, the OS and PFS were comparable. When evaluating samples in 15 patients for allelic fraction (AF) and separating patients along the median value into high and low AF, differences were observed, which may convey a prognostic value. Patients with low AF showed an OS of 552 days compared with high AF, which showed an OS of 411 days. PFS differences were not statistically significant.[8]

Ceritinib

With positive results in the use of crizotinib in ROS1-mutated NSCLC, ceritinib, as the initial second-generation ALK inhibitor with proven benefit in crizotinib-naive and crizotinib-treated patients with ALK-mutated NSCLC, was investigated for its utility in ROS1-mutated NSCLC given ceritinib's ability to inhibit ROS1 in vitro. A phase II study of 32 patients with ROS1-rearranged NSCLC who had progressed on standard therapy was conducted using ceritinib 750 mg by mouth daily. Thirty of the 32 patients were crizotinib naive and the 2 patients who had progressed on crizotinib were not evaluable because of progression or death. When taking the cohort altogether, the ORR was 62%, the DCR was 81%, and the median PFS was 9.3 months. When excluding the 2 crizotinib pretreated patients, the ORR improved to 67%, the DCR to 87%, and the median PFS to 19.3 months. The median OS was 24 months with a 12-month OS of 56%. In addition, intracranial ORR was 25% and DCR was 63% in patients with baseline central nervous system (CNS) metastases. This trial showed favorable outcome data in crizotinib-naive patients with ROS1-rearranged NSCLC; however, it indicated a low likelihood of response in patients previously treated with crizotinib, although the sample size was miniscule. In addition, side effects, namely gastrointestinal (GI) toxicity including diarrhea and nausea, were higher with ceritinib, raising questions of tolerability, with 68% of patients requiring dose adjustments and 72% requiring dose interruption.[34]

Lorlatinib

Lorlatinib, a highly selective third-generation ALK and ROS1 TKI, is approved as second-line therapy for patients with ALK-positive NSCLC given retained potency against secondary ALK resistance mutations. Compared with crizotinib, ceritinib, alectinib, and foretinib in vitro, lorlatinib shows at least a 10-fold improved potency against ROS1. In addition, in vitro data support retained activity of lorlatinib against ROS1 G2032R and L2026M secondary resistance mutations.[35] In the phase I study of lorlatinib in patients with ALK fusion–positive or ROS1 fusion–positive locally advanced or metastatic NSCLC, 54 patients were evaluable. Among those, 12 harbored ROS1 fusion with 7 patients previously receiving ROS1 targeted TKIs. For this group, the ORR was 50% with a DCR of 67% and an overall PFS of 7.0 months. The intracranial ORR was 3 of 5 patients (60%). The recommended phase 2 dose was 100 mg by mouth daily.[36]

The phase I/II expansion of lorlatinib treatment of ROS1 fusion–positive NSCLC is currently ongoing, with 59 patients enrolled with 51 tumor samples evaluable. Thirty-eight patients previously received ROS1-targeted TKIs, with G2032R being the most frequent secondary resistance mutation with an ORR of 29.4%. Among patients previously treated with TKIs, the ORR was 23.8% if no secondary mutation was found and 33.3% if a secondary resistance mutation was found. Of patients with the G2032R secondary mutation, all had stable disease. Thirteen patients were ROS1 TKI naive and had an ORR of 76.9%.[37]

Entrectinib

The multitargeted TKI entrectinib, for ALK, ROS1, and NTRK1/2/3, has shown promising results for the treatment of ROS1-mutated NSCLC and shows a potency for ROS1 30 times stronger than crizotinib.[38] Data from 2 phase I studies, ALKA-372-001 and STARTRK-1, were compiled providing efficacy data. These studies enrolled 119 patients with advanced solid tumors who had previously received at least 3 lines of therapy (including 27% of patients receiving previous ALK or ROS1 TKIs) for their malignancies with any type of alteration in ALK, ROS1, or NTRK1/2/3 allowed. Responses were only observed in patients who harbored gene fusions and not in those with amplifications, copy number variants, insertions, or deletions. In addition, patients with ALK or ROS1 fusion who previously progressed on targeted TKIs did not show favorable responses. Two dose-limiting toxicities were observed at the 800-mg by mouth daily dose level and thus 600 mg by mouth daily was chosen as the recommended phase 2 dose.[39]

An analysis was performed on the phase II eligible population, which included patients with ALK, ROS1, or NTRK1/2/3 fusions who had never received ALK/ROS1 TKIs and who were exposed to doses equivalent to 600 mg by mouth daily. Of these patients, 14 had ROS1-rearranged solid tumors, 13 of which were NSCLC. Within this subgroup, the ORR was 86% with 2 complete responses. Median PFS was 19.0 months with 1 patient with continued response at 32 months at data analysis. In addition, 8 patients with ALK, ROS1, or NTRK1/2/3 mutations in the phase II eligible population had brain metastases, with a response in 63% of patients, showing penetration through the blood-brain barrier.[39]

An abstract reporting the results for ROS1 fusion–positive NSCLC from a pooled analysis of the phase I studies discussed earlier (ALKA-372-001 and STARTRK-1) in addition to the ongoing phase II study STARTRK-2, which enrolled locally advanced or metastatic ALK, ROS1, or NTRK1/2/3 fusion solid tumors and only allowed prior treatment with crizotinib in NSCLC with brain-only recurrence, was presented at AACR (American Association for Cancer Research) 2019. Of the patients enrolled, there were 53 TKI-naive patients with ROS1 fusion–positive NSCLC. The reported ORR was 77% with 3 complete responses. PFS was 26 months for patients without CNS disease and 14 months for patients with CNS disease at baseline. Intracranial ORR was 55%.[40]

Repotrectinib

Repotrectinib, a next-generation ALK, ROS1, and NTRK1/2/3 fusion inhibitor, is also under investigation for the treatment of ROS1 fusion-positive NSCLC. Although entrectinib seems to have limited utility in the setting of previous ROS1 TKI use, preclinical data indicate activity of repotrectinib against secondary solvent front mutations in ROS1, namely G2032R and D2033N, as well as theorized effective CNS penetration.[41] In the phase I clinical trial TRIDENT-1, enrolling patients with locally advanced or metastatic solid tumors positive for ALK, ROS1, or NTRK1/2/3 fusion, 31 ROS1 fusion–positive tumors (29 NSCLC) were evaluable under different dose escalation cohorts. The ORR was 70% among TKI-naive patients and 11% among TKI-refractory patients, with a patient with CD74-ROS1 NSCLC with brain metastases and confirmed G2032R secondary mutation showing a partial response, including in the CNS.[42]

DS-6051b

DS-6051b is a TKI developed with a high affinity for both ROS1 and NTRK1/2/3. Both in vitro and in vivo mice xenograft models showed affinity of DS-6051b for wild-type ROS1 as well as G2032R-mutated ROS1 with DS-6015b more effectively inhibiting G2032R tumor xenograft growth than lorlatinib.[43] The US phase I study of DS-6051b in advanced solid tumors with either ROS1 or NTRK [Neurotrophic Tropomyosin Receptor Kinase] fusions enrolled 9 patients with ROS1 fusions, 7 of whom were previously treated with ROS1 TKIs. Of the 6 evaluable patients, all were previously treated with crizotinib and showed an ORR of 33.3% and DCR of 66.7%. The maximum tolerated dose was 800 mg by mouth daily.[44]

In a Japanese phase I study of DS-6051b in advanced ROS1 fusion–positive NSCLC, 15 patients were enrolled. Twelve of the patients had measurable disease and 9 of the 12 were ROS1 TKI naive. The ORR was 58.3% for the overall cohort, 66.7% in TKI-naive patients, and 33.3% in TKI-pretreated patients, whereas the DCR was 100% overall. The recommended phase 2 dose was determined to be 600 mg by mouth daily. The discrepancy between the US and Japanese phase I trials can be ascribed to an increased area under the curve in Japanese patients on 800 mg by mouth daily, which decreased when corrected for body weight, indicating a likely consequence of different median weights for patients in the United States and Japan.[45] **Table 1** provides a summary of the numerous studies discussed evaluating TKI efficacy in ROS1-rearranged NSCLC.

ROS1 RESISTANCE MECHANISMS

ROS1-rearranged NSCLC is an oncogene-addicted malignancy that depends on

Table 1
Summary of clinical trials using different tyrosine kinase inhibitors in ROS1-rearranged non-small cell lung cancer

Drug	Study	Phase	Patients (N)	ORR (%)	DCR (%)	mPFS (mo)	mOS (mo)
Crizotinib	PROFILE 1001	Prospective I/II	50	72	90	19.3	51.4
	EUROS1	Retrospective	31	80	86.6	9.1	NA
	East Asian	Prospective II	127	71.7	88.2	15.9	12-mo 83.1%[a]
	EUCROSS	Prospective II	18	83	NA	NA	NA
	AcSé	Prospective II	37	71	85	10	NA
	Shanghai	Retrospective	49	83.3	97.2	12.6	32.7
Ceritinib	—	Prospective II	30[b]	67	87	19.3	24
Lorlatinib	—	Prospective I	12[c]	50	67	7	NA
Entrectinib	ALKA-372-001 & STARTRK1	Prospective I/II	14	86	NA	19.0	NA
Repotrectinib	TRIDENT-1	Prospective I	29[c]	31	NA	NA	NA
DS-6051b	United States	Prospective I	6[c]	33.3	66.7	NA	NA
	Japan	Prospective I	12[c]	58.3	100	NA	NA

Abbreviations: mOS, median OS; mPFS, median PFS; NA, not available or not reached; ORR, objective response rate. DCR, disease control rate.

[a] 83.1% of patients survived at least 12 months.

[b] Data exclude crizotinib-resistant patients.

[c] Data include both crizotinib-naive and crizotinib-resistant patients.

upregulation of ROS1 and resultant activation of downstream regulators to proliferate and survive. On exposure to ROS1 TKIs, tumor cells undergo apoptosis or transition to a quiescent state and eventually develop resistance mechanisms to reproliferate even in the setting of targeted TKIs. Resistance through pharmacokinetic abnormalities of poor compliance, poor absorption through the GI tract, differences in enzymatic metabolism, and differences in blood-brain barrier penetration should always be considered; however, resistance in those adequately exposed to targeted TKIs is discussed here.[46]

ROS1-dependent Mechanism of Resistance: Secondary Mutations

TKIs used in the treatment of ROS1 fusion–positive NSCLC act to block the constitutive activation of the ROS1 kinase via linkage to fusion partners by competitively binding in the ATP-binding pocket. Secondary mutations affecting the ROS1-binding pocket are often point mutations leading to a single amino acid substitution, with different sized or charged amino acids weakening or blocking binding of small molecule TKIs. Ultimately this leads to decreased binding of TKIs and allows the activation of downstream regulators to promote proliferation.

The gatekeeper residue is often the site of a critical amino acid within the ATP-binding pocket that, when mutated, affects TKI affinity. In EGFR-mutated lung cancer, the T790M mutation is the gatekeeper mutation and is implicated in most resistance to first-generation and second-generation EGFR TKIs, estimated at 50% to 65% of secondary mutations. In contrast, the ROS1 gatekeeper residue L2026M, like the ALK gatekeeper residue of L1196M, only accounts for a fraction of secondary mutations.[35,46] Clinically, the ROS1 L2026M mutation is rarely seen, although in vitro studies have indicated that cell lines with L2026M mutations were resistant to crizotinib but sensitive to both ceritinib and lorlatinib.[35,47]

The first published case of a secondary mutation was identified in a postcrizotinib progression sample of a patient with CD74-ROS1 fusion NSCLC. The G2032R ROS1 mutation exists at the solvent front region at the distal end of the kinase hinge, blocking binding of crizotinib but still allowing ATP binding, and is analogous to the G1202R ALK resistance mutation. In this patient an autopsy was performed and it was determined that all sites of disease carried the G2032R mutation, likely indicating the presence of G2032R ROS1 in small founder clones that emerged under the pressure of crizotinib treatment.[48] CD74-ROS1 fusion cells with G2032R were created in vitro and were found to be highly resistant to treatment with either crizotinib or ceritinib. However, cabozantinib, a multikinase VEGFR, RET, MET, AXL, and ROS1 inhibitor, effectively inhibited the growth and phosphorylation of downstream signals in these cells. When tested on a cell line of CD74-ROS1 G2032R created from the pleural effusion of a patient who progressed on crizotinib, cabozantinib effectively inhibited growth.[47] As discussed previously, preclinical and clinical evidence indicate at least partial sensitivity of G2032R to lorlatinib and repotrectinib.[35,37,41]

The D2033N mutation exists at the solvent front region of the ATP-binding pocket and was identified in a patient with CD74-ROS1 NSCLC who progressed after crizotinib therapy and is analogous to the D1203N ALK resistance mutation. In this case, the patient was successfully treated with cabozantinib, showing a near-complete response, and remained on therapy for at least 8 months at the time of publication. In vitro, CD74-ROS1 D2033N cells showed resistance to crizotinib, ceritinib, brigatinib, and lorlatinib, but remained susceptible to cabozantinib and foretinib.[49] Preclinical evidence also suggests the utility of repotrectinib in the treatment of D2033N-mutated ROS1 NSCLC.[41]

The S1986Y/F mutations occur outside the kinase-binding pocket and instead affect the αC helix, altering the conformation of the pocket. The mutations were identified in a patient with EZR-ROS1 NSCLC after crizotinib therapy, and are analogous to the C1156Y ALK resistance mutation. Clinically, the patient was treated with lorlatinib with an excellent response and remained on therapy for at least 6 months at data analysis. In vitro, S1986F EZR-ROS1 and S1986Y EZR-ROS1 cells were evaluated and noted to be resistant to crizotinib and ceritinib, but they were sensitive to lorlatinib with an associated decrease in phosphorylation of downstream signaling.[50]

The incidence of these secondary resistance mutations was evaluated in a retrospective analysis of patients with ROS1 fusion NSCLC who progressed after crizotinib therapy. In a cohort of 17, 53% of specimens were found to have secondary resistance mutations, with 41% containing G2032R, 6% with D2033N, and 6% with S1986F. None of the 3 evaluable patients with CNS disease developed secondary mutations and although this sample size is small, the lack of secondary mutations may be explained by the inability of crizotinib to effectively penetrate the blood-brain barrier.[51]

Given the homology of ROS1 and ALK kinase domains to each other, especially with evidence in L2026M, G2032R, D2033N, and S1986Y/F of corresponding ALK mutations and similar resistance profiles, secondary ROS1 mutations not yet seen clinically were theorized. The corresponding ALK to ROS1 mutation suppositions are as follows: 1151Tins to 1981Tins, L1152R to L1982F, I1171T to M2001T, F1174C/V to F2004C/V, and G1269A to G2101A.[50] In addition, an L2155S secondary ROS1 mutation, which would be analogous to ALK F1323 (although never described) was identified in vitro in SLC34A2-ROS1 cells causing protein structural malformation and leading to modification of the crizotinib-binding site. This mutation showed resistance to crizotinib and foretinib.[52] **Table 2** contains a list of clinically relevant secondary ROS1 NSCLC mutations published.

ROS1-independent Mechanism of Resistance: Bypass Signaling Pathways

Although secondary ROS1 mutations attempt to alter the binding of inhibitors and allow constitutive activation of the ROS1 pathway, resistance can also develop via the subversion of the ROS1 pathway in favor of an alternative bypass pathway that can independently phosphorylate downstream signaling and lead to cell proliferation.

The development of constitutive activation of the EGFR pathway can decrease the need for dependence on the original ROS1 oncogenic driver. Treatment of SLC34A2-ROS1 cells with TAE684, a selective ROS1 inhibitor with few off-target effects, led to the eventual development of

Table 2
Clinically applicable ROS1 secondary mutations with respective anaplastic lymphoma kinase–rearranged non–small cell lung cancer analogues as well as tyrosine kinase inhibitors likely able to produce a response

Resistance Mutation	Mutation Type	Effective Treatments	ALK Analogue
L2026M	Gatekeeper	Ceritinib, lorlatinib	L1196M
G2032R	Solvent front	Cabozantinib, lorlatinib, repotrectinib	G1202R
D2033N	Solvent front	Cabozantinib, repotrectinib	D1203N
S1986Y/F	αC helix	Lorlatinib	C1156Y

cells that could survive in media with TAE684. Analysis of these cells found no secondary ROS1 mutations or driver mutations and, although ROS1 and SHP-2 phosphorylation were decreased, both ERK1/2 and AKT phosphorylation were stable to increased compared with controls. In addition, EGFR phosphorylation was maintained and MET phosphorylation was decreased. When these cells were exposed to different EGFR inhibitors, there was a modest decrease in cellular proliferation; however, the addition of TAE684 with an EGFR inhibitor further sensitized the cells to the inhibitory effects.[53]

A second in vitro analysis showed similar results in a SLC34A2-ROS1 cell line with crizotinib resistance showing no secondary ROS1 mutations; however, increased EGFR signaling was detected, with the most effective inhibition of signaling observed with the combination of ROS1 and EGFR inhibitors.[52] In addition, a cell line derived from a CD74-ROS1 postcrizotinib progression patient sample without detectable mutations was found to have retained HER2 expression and phosphorylation. The addition of afatinib to crizotinib partially inhibited cell proliferation as well as downstream AKT and ERK1/2 signaling.[54]

A second bypass pathway through the RAS pathway has been described. Resistance to ROS1 inhibitors was generated in SLC34A2-ROS1 NSCLC cells with decreased ROS1 phosphorylation at the same time as phosphorylation levels of AKT, mitogen-activated protein kinase (MAPK), and S6 kinase were maintained or improved. Two populations of cells, 1 with a KRAS G12C mutation and the other with an NRAS Q61K mutation, were created. Both showed resistance to crizotinib but developed renewed sensitivity to crizotinib when treated with MAPK and AKT inhibitors or when the respective KRAS or NRAS mutations were silenced. Tumor samples from 4 patients with NSCLC who progressed on crizotinib were collected, with 1 showing KRAS amplification, which may have contributed to resistance.[55] In a separate study, a cell line created from exposure of SLC34A2-ROS1 NSCLC cells to entrectinib was created. Secondary ROS1 mutations were not found; however, the KRAS G12C mutation was detected and suspected as the driving resistance mechanism. Although selumetinib, a mitogen-activated protein kinase kinase (MEK) inhibitor, alone was able to minimally inhibit these entrectinib-resistant cells, the combination of selumetinib and entrectinib completely inhibited ERK phosphorylation and significantly, although not completely, inhibited cellular growth.[56]

In addition, KIT mutations have been implicated in creating bypass signaling pathways. The KIT D816G mutation was identified in a tumor sample of a patient with ROS1-positive NSCLC with detectable mRNA of KIT in the postcrizotinib progression sample, but not before treatment. To evaluate this pathway further, KIT D816G was added to ROS1-positive cell lines. The addition of ponatinib, an inhibitor of KIT D816G, to crizotinib maximally inhibited AKT and ERK1/2 compared with either alone.[57] A separate analysis of ROS1 postcrizotinib progression samples identified a sample with KIT D816G mutation thought to be driving resistance.[54]

SUMMARY

Identifying ROS1-rearranged NSCLC is important in order to appropriately treat these patients with crizotinib or entrectinib, with multiple other TKIs being studied in this setting. Postprogression biopsies are necessary to identify potential resistance mechanisms and are important in choosing second-line therapies, whether with a subsequent TKI, such as lorlatinib or cabozantinib, or transitioning to a chemotherapy and immunotherapy–based approach.

DISCLOSURE

LB has received advisory board honoraria from the following companies in the past 12 months: Blueprint, Takeda, Astra Zeneca, Genentech, BeyondSpring Pharmaceuticals, G1 Therapeutics, Boehringer Ingelheim.

REFERENCES

1. Rimkunas VM, Crosby KE, Li D, et al. Analysis of receptor tyrosine kinase ROS1-positive tumors in non-small cell lung cancer: identification of a FIG-ROS1 fusion. Clin Cancer Res 2012;18(16):4449–57.
2. Gainor JF, Shaw AT. Novel targets in non-small cell lung cancer: ROS1 and RET fusions. Oncologist 2013;18(7):865–75.
3. Shibuya M, Hanafusa H, Balduzzi PC. Cellular sequences related to three new onc genes of avian sarcoma virus (fps, yes, and ros) and their expression in normal and transformed cells. J Virol 1982;42(1):143–52.
4. Matsushime H, Wang LH, Shibuya M. Human c-ros-1 gene homologous to the v-ros sequence of UR2 sarcoma virus encodes for a transmembrane receptorlike molecule. Mol Cell Biol 1986;6(8):3000–4.
5. Sharma S, Birchmeier C, Nikawa J, et al. Characterization of the ros1-gene products expressed in human glioblastoma cell lines. Oncogene Res 1989;5(2):91–100.
6. Roskoski R Jr. ROS1 protein-tyrosine kinase inhibitors in the treatment of ROS1 fusion protein-driven

non-small cell lung cancers. Pharmacol Res 2017; 121:202–12.
7. Charest A, Lane K, McMahon K, et al. Fusion of FIG to the receptor tyrosine kinase ROS in a glioblastoma with an interstitial del(6)(q21q21). Genes Chromosomes Cancer 2003;37(1):58–71.
8. He Y, Sheng W, Hu W, et al. Different types of ROS1 fusion partners yield comparable efficacy to crizotinib. Oncol Res 2019;27(8):901–10.
9. Davies KD, Le AT, Theodoro MF, et al. Identifying and targeting ROS1 gene fusions in non-small cell lung cancer. Clin Cancer Res 2012;18(17):4570–9.
10. Gu TL, Deng X, Huang F, et al. Survey of tyrosine kinase signaling reveals ROS kinase fusions in human cholangiocarcinoma. PLoS One 2011;6(1):e15640.
11. Charest A, Wilker EW, McLaughlin ME, et al. ROS fusion tyrosine kinase activates a SH2 domain-containing phosphatase-2/phosphatidylinositol 3-kinase/mammalian target of rapamycin signaling axis to form glioblastoma in mice. Cancer Res 2006;66(15):7473–81.
12. Ou SH, Tan J, Yen Y, et al. ROS1 as a 'druggable' receptor tyrosine kinase: lessons learned from inhibiting the ALK pathway. Expert Rev Anticancer Ther 2012;12(4):447–56.
13. Huber KV, Salah E, Radic B, et al. Stereospecific targeting of MTH1 by (S)-crizotinib as an anticancer strategy. Nature 2014;508(7495):222–7.
14. Bubendorf L, Buttner R, Al-Dayel F, et al. Testing for ROS1 in non-small cell lung cancer: a review with recommendations. Virchows Arch 2016;469(5): 489–503.
15. Cao B, Wei P, Liu Z, et al. Detection of lung adenocarcinoma with ROS1 rearrangement by IHC, FISH, and RT-PCR and analysis of its clinicopathologic features. Onco Targets Ther 2016;9:131–8.
16. Lindeman NI, Cagle PT, Aisner DL, et al. Updated molecular testing guideline for the selection of lung cancer patients for treatment with targeted tyrosine kinase inhibitors: guideline from the College of American Pathologists, the International Association for the Study of Lung Cancer, and the Association for Molecular Pathology. J Thorac Oncol 2018;13(3):323–58.
17. Sholl LM, Sun H, Butaney M, et al. ROS1 immunohistochemistry for detection of ROS1-rearranged lung adenocarcinomas. Am J Surg Pathol 2013;37(9): 1441–9.
18. Yoshida A, Tsuta K, Wakai S, et al. Immunohistochemical detection of ROS1 is useful for identifying ROS1 rearrangements in lung cancers. Mod Pathol 2014;27(5):711–20.
19. Su Y, Goncalves T, Dias-Santagata D, et al. Immunohistochemical Detection of ROS1 Fusion. Am J Clin Pathol 2017;147(1):77–82.
20. Shan L, Lian F, Guo L, et al. Detection of ROS1 gene rearrangement in lung adenocarcinoma: comparison of IHC, FISH and real-time RT-PCR. PLoS One 2015; 10(3):e0120422.
21. Cha YJ, Lee JS, Kim HR, et al. Screening of ROS1 rearrangements in lung adenocarcinoma by immunohistochemistry and comparison with ALK rearrangements. PLoS One 2014;9(7):e103333.
22. Zheng Z, Liebers M, Zhelyazhova B, et al. Anchored multiplex PCR for targeted next-generation sequencing. Nat Med 2014;20(12):1479–84.
23. Zhang L, Jiang T, Zhao C, et al. Efficacy of crizotinib and pemetrexed-based chemotherapy in Chinese NSCLC patients with ROS1 rearrangement. Oncotarget 2016;7(46):75145–54.
24. Shaw AT, Varghese AM, Solomon BJ, et al. Pemetrexed-based chemotherapy in patients with advanced, ALK-positive non-small cell lung cancer. Ann Oncol 2013;24(1):59–66.
25. Chen YF, Hsieh MS, Wu SG, et al. Efficacy of pemetrexed-based chemotherapy in patients with ROS1 fusion-positive lung adenocarcinoma compared with in patients harboring other driver mutations in East Asian populations. J Thorac Oncol 2016;11(7):1140–52.
26. Kwak EL, Camidge DR, Clark JW, et al. Clinical activity observed in a phase I dose escalation trial of an oral c-MET and ALK inhibitor, PF-02341066. J Clin Oncol 2009;27:3509 [abstract].
27. Shaw AT, Ou SH, Bang YJ, et al. Crizotinib in ROS1-rearranged non-small-cell lung cancer. N Engl J Med 2014;371(21):1963–71.
28. Shaw AT, Riely GJ, Bang YJ, et al. Crizotinib in ROS1-rearranged advanced non-small-cell lung cancer (NSCLC): updated results, including overall survival, from PROFILE 1001. Ann Oncol 2019; 30(7):1121–6.
29. Mazières J, Zalcman G, Crinò L, et al. Crizotinib therapy for advanced lung adenocarcinoma and a ROS1 rearrangement: results from the EUROS1 cohort. J Clin Oncol 2015;33(9):992–9.
30. Wu YL, Yang JC, Kim DW, et al. Phase II study of crizotinib in East Asian patients with ROS1-positive advanced non-small-cell lung cancer. J Clin Oncol 2018;36(14):1405–11.
31. Moro-Sibilot D, Faivre L, Zalcman G, et al. Crizotinib in patients with advanced ROS1 rearranged non-small cell lung cancer (NSCLC): preliminary results of the AcSé phase II trial. J Clin Oncol 2015;33:8065.
32. Michels S, Gardizi M, Schmalz P, et al. EUCROSS: a European phase II trial of crizotinib in advanced adenocarcinoma of the lung harboring ROS1 rearrangements - preliminary results. J Thorac Oncol 2017;12(1):S379–80 [abstract].
33. Li Z, Shen L, Ding D, et al. Efficacy of crizotinib among different types of ROS1 fusion partners in patients with ROS1-rearranged non-small cell lung cancer. J Thorac Oncol 2018;13(7):987–95.

34. Lim SM, Kim HR, Lee JS, et al. Open-label, multicenter, phase II study of ceritinib in patients with non-small-cell lung cancer harboring ROS1 rearrangement. J Clin Oncol 2017;35(23):2613–8.
35. Zou HY, Li Q, Engstrom LD, et al. PF-06463922 is a potent and selective next-generation ROS1/ALK inhibitor capable of blocking crizotinib-resistant ROS1 mutations. Proc Natl Acad Sci U S A 2015; 112(11):3493–8.
36. Shaw AT, Felip E, Bauer TM, et al. Lorlatinib in non-small-cell lung cancer with ALK or ROS1 rearrangement: an international, multicentre, open-label, single-arm first-in-man phase 1 trial. Lancet Oncol 2017;18(12):1590–9.
37. Solomon BJ, Martini JF, Ou SH, et al. Efficacy of lorlatinib in patients (pts) with ROS1-positive advanced non-small cell lung cancer (NSCLC) and ROS1 kinase domain mutations. Ann Oncol 2018;29: 1380PD [abstract].
38. Doebele R, Ahn M, Siena S, et al. Efficacy and safety of entrectinib in locally advanced or metastatic ROS1 fusion-positive non-small cell lung cancer (NSCLC). J Thorac Oncol 2018;13(10):S321–2 [abstract].
39. Drilon A, Siena S, Ou SI, et al. Safety and antitumor activity of the multitargeted pan-TRK, ROS1, and ALK inhibitor entrectinib: combined results from two phase I trials (ALKA-372-001 and STARTRK-1). Cancer Discov 2017;7(4):400–9.
40. Drilon A, Barlesi F, De Braud FG, et al. Entrectinib in locally advanced or metastatic ROS1 fusion-positive non-small cell lung cancer (NSCLC): integrated analysis of ALKA-372-001, STARTRK-1 and STARTRK-2. Proceedings of the AACR Annual Meeting. Geneva, Switzerland, April 10–13, 2019.
41. Drilon A, Ou SI, Cho BC, et al. Repotrectinib (TPX-0005) is a next-generation ROS1/TRK/ALK inhibitor that potently inhibits ROS1/TRK/ALK solvent- front mutations. Cancer Discov 2018;8(10):1227–36.
42. Drilon A, Ou SI, Cho BC, et al. A phase 1 study of the next-generation ALK/ROS1/TRK inhibitor ropotrectinib (TPX-0005) in patients with advanced ALK/ ROS1/NTRK+ cancers (TRIDENT-1). J Clin Oncol 2018;36:2513.
43. Katayama R, Gong B, Togashi N, et al. The new-generation selective ROS1/NTRK inhibitor DS-6051b overcomes crizotinib resistant ROS1-G2032R mutation in preclinical models. Nat Commun 2019;10(1):3604.
44. Papdopoulos KP, Gandhi L, Janne PA, et al. First-in-human study of DS-6051b in patients (pts) with advanced solid tumors (AST) conducted in the US. J Clin Oncol 2018;36:2514 [abstract].
45. Fujiwara Y, Takeda M, Yamamoto N, et al. Safety and pharmacokinetics of DS-6051b in Japanese patients with non-small cell lung cancer harboring ROS1 fusions: a phase I study. Oncotarget 2018;9(34): 23729–37.
46. Camidge DR, Pao W, Sequist LV. Acquired resistance to TKIs in solid tumours: learning from lung cancer. Nat Rev Clin Oncol 2014;11(8):473–81.
47. Katayama R, Kobayashi Y, Friboulet L, et al. Cabozantinib overcomes crizotinib resistance in ROS1 fusion-positive cancer. Clin Cancer Res 2015;21(1): 166–74.
48. Awad MM, Katayama R, McTigue M, et al. Acquired resistance to crizotinib from a mutation in CD74-ROS1. N Engl J Med 2013;368(25):2395–401.
49. Drilon A, Somwar R, Wagner JP, et al. A novel crizotinib-resistant solvent-front mutation responsive to cabozantinib therapy in a patient with ROS1-rearranged lung cancer. Clin Cancer Res 2016; 22(10):2351–8.
50. Facchinetti F, Loriot Y, Kuo MS, et al. Crizotinib-resistant ROS1 mutations reveal a predictive kinase inhibitor sensitivity model for ROS1- and ALK-rearranged lung cancers. Clin Cancer Res 2016; 22(24):5983–91.
51. Gainor JK, Tseng D, Yoda S, et al. Patterns of metastatic spread and mechanisms of resistance to crizotinib in ROS1-positive non-small-cell lung cancer. JCO Precis Oncol 2017;2017:1–19.
52. Song A, Kim TM, Kim DW, et al. Molecular changes associated with acquired resistance to crizotinib in ROS1-rearranged non-small cell lung cancer. Clin Cancer Res 2015;21(10):2379–87.
53. Davies KD, Mahale S, Astling DP, et al. Resistance to ROS1 inhibition mediated by EGFR pathway activation in non-small cell lung cancer. PLoS One 2013; 8(12):e82236.
54. McCoach CE, Le AT, Gowan K, et al. Resistance mechanisms to targeted therapies in ROS1(+) and ALK(+) non-small cell lung cancer. Clin Cancer Res 2018;24(14):3334–47.
55. Cargnelutti M, Corso S, Pergolizzi M, et al. Activation of RAS family members confers resistance to ROS1 targeting drugs. Oncotarget 2015;6(7):5182–94.
56. Ku BM, Bae YH, Lee KY, et al. Entrectinib resistance mechanisms in ROS1-rearranged non-small cell lung cancer. Invest New Drugs 2019. [Epub ahead of print].
57. Dziadziuszko R, Le AT, Wrona A, et al. An activating KIT mutation induces crizotinib resistance in ROS1-positive lung cancer. J Thorac Oncol 2016;11(8): 1273–81.

Molecular Targets Beyond the Big 3

Karen L. Reckamp, MD, MS

KEYWORDS

• Targeted therapy • Gene mutations • BRAF • NTRK • KRAS • MET • RET • HER2

KEY POINTS

- Targeted therapies have improved outcomes in patients whose tumors have oncogenic driver alterations.
- Understanding these genetic alterations and mechanisms of resistance in non-small cell lung cancer will expand our ability to treat patients and extend their survival.
- Precision medicine is a reality as tumor genotyping becomes increasingly accessible and will continue to transform as sequencing technology evolves.
- Genetic alterations in *BRAF* and *NTRK* are uncommon in non-small cell lung cancer but have associated approved targeted therapies which result in tumor response and better outcomes for patients.
- Additional genomic alterations are identified and under investigation; some of the most promising with targeted therapies in clinical trials include ***KRAS, MET, RET, HER2, and NRG***.

INTRODUCTION

Lung cancer is a heterogeneous genomic disease.[1] Although smoking remains the primary cause of lung cancer, genetic susceptibility and environmental exposures are responsible for 10% to 15% of cases.[2] Targeted therapies improved survival in patients with tumors with oncogenic drivers.[3] Therefore, it is critical to expand our understanding of genetic alterations in non-small cell lung cancer (NSCLC) to increase the number of targeted therapies available for patients. Alterations beyond epidermal growth factor receptor (*EGFR*), *ALK*, and *ROS1* exemplify lung cancer's complexity and the need for greater investments in precision therapy to extend patient survival and outcomes. This article covers genetic targets outside of the big 3 (*BRAF*, *NTRK*, *KRAS*, *HER2*, *RET*, *MET*, *NRG1*), their novel agents, challenges, and future directions.

B-RAF PROTO-ONCOGENE

The *BRAF* proto-oncogene encodes for the serine/threonine kinase that lies downstream of *rat sarcoma* (*RAS*) and leads to signaling through the RAS-rapidly accelerated fibrosarcoma (RAF)-mitogen-activated protein kinase (MAPK)-MAPK/extracellular-signal-regulated kinase (ERK) (MEK)-ERK signaling pathways, a key molecular cascade that regulates cell growth.[4] After *BRAF* mutations were first described in melanoma, mutant *BRAF* was shown to mediate oncogenesis in lung adenocarcinoma.[5] *BRAF* mutations represent 2% to 3% of lung adenocarcinomas, with 50% to 75% *BRAF* V600 E, and more frequently found in patients with a tobacco use history.[6,7]

Vemurafenib demonstrated efficacy in patients with *BRAF* V600 E mutated metastatic NSCLC.[8,9] Dabrafenib was evaluated in a phase II trial in patients with metastatic *BRAF* V600 E mutant

Cedars-Sinai Medical Center, 8700 Beverly Boulevard, Los Angeles, CA 90048, USA
E-mail address: karen.reckamp@cshs.org

Thorac Surg Clin 30 (2020) 157–164
https://doi.org/10.1016/j.thorsurg.2020.01.004
1547-4127/20/

NSCLC.[10] The overall response rate (ORR) was 33%, and the median overall survival (OS) was 12.7 months. A combination of dabrafenib and trametinib was studied in another phase II trial of patients with *BRAF* V600 E mutant NSCLC.[10] The combination therapy resulted in an increased ORR (63.2%) and has been approved by the European Medicines Agency and the US Food and Drug Administration for patients with stage IV NSCLC with *BRAF* V600 E mutation.

NEUROTROPHIN TYROSINE KINASE RECEPTOR

Tropomyosin-related kinase (*TRK*) encodes the tyrosine kinase receptors for neurotrophins found in multiple tissues and associated with the nerve growth factor family.[11] Three members of the family are proto-oncogenes encoded by *NTRK1*, *NTRK2*, and *NTRK3*, which produce the proteins TrkA, TrkB, and TrkC, respectively, and activation leads to signaling in the MAPK and AKT pathways among others leading to cell proliferation, differentiation, and survival.[12] Neurotrophin tyrosine kinase receptor (*NTRK*) rearrangements can occur in all 3 genes and have been identified in multiple cancers, including lung cancer.[13] Fewer than 1% of NSCLC cases have *NTRK* fusions. *NTRK* fusions are found in men and women with various ages and smoking histories.[14]

Multiple tyrosine kinase inhibitors (TKI) are being investigated for *NTRK*-altered cancers. The US Food and Drug Administration granted larotrectinib and entrectinib accelerated approval for adult and pediatric solid tumors positive for *NTRK* fusions, which will be the focus of the clinical data presented. The first patient with *NTRK* fusion to demonstrate tumor regression with a selective TRK inhibitor, larotrectinib, was reported in 2015; preclinical models confirmed tumor growth inhibition.[15] A phase I trial investigated larotrectinib in adult and pediatric patients with *NTRK* fusions across tumor types. In the 55 patients enrolled across 13 tumor types, the most common fusions observed were *NTRK3* (n = 29), followed by *NTRK1* (n = 25) and *NTRK2* (n = 1), with 14 unique fusion partners.[16] The study demonstrated a 75% ORR in *NTRK* fusion-positive patients.

Early results from an entrectinib phase I study reported antitumor activity in a patient with an *NTRK1* fusion NSCLC.[17] An analysis of 3 early phase trials investigating entrectinib with *NTRK* or *ROS1* positive tumors enrolled 54 patients with *NTRK* fusions with a 57% ORR.[18] The median progression-free survival (PFS) was 11.2 months, and OS was 20.9 months. Additional TRK inhibitors are under investigation in the clinic.

KIRSTEN RAT SARCOMA VIRAL ONCOGENE

Kirsten RAS viral oncogene (*KRAS*) is the most commonly mutated of the *RAS* family isoforms and occurs in 22% of tumors, one of the most common oncogenic driver mutations in cancer.[19] Most *KRAS* mutations are found in exons 12 and 13 (39% G12C, 18%–21% G12V, and 17%–18% G12D).[20] In advanced NSCLC, *KRAS* mutation is associated with poorer prognosis.[21] Despite its early discovery, *KRAS*-mutant NSCLC is highly heterogeneous, and therapy targeting *KRAS* is just beginning to be understood.

KRAS is 1 of the 4 proteins encoded by *RAS*. Guanosine triphosphate binds to KRAS in the active state and guanosine diphosphate binds to KRAS in the inactive state (**Fig. 1**A). Activating point mutations in RAS proteins like KRAS typically confer tumorigenesis by loss of GTPase activity; this results in the active state and constitutive activation of downstream signaling pathways like phosphatidylinositol 3-kinase (PI3K) and MAPK, rendering them resistant to multiple standard therapies for NSCLC (**Fig. 1**B).[22]

Previous attempts to target KRAS failed due to a lack of known allosteric binding sites, alternative pathways, and the protein's high affinity for the active guanosine triphosphate–bound state.[23,24] Other attempts included combination therapy with MAPK kinase (MEK1/MEK2) inhibition. A phase II clinical trial in advanced *KRAS*-mutant NSCLC demonstrated efficacy at the cost of high toxicity. The selumetinib-docetaxel combination resulted in a 37% increase in ORR and 3.2-month PFS compared with patients who received docetaxel. The combination group experienced a 15% increase in grade 3 adverse events (AEs) with the most common grade 3 of 4 AEs being neutropenia, febrile neutropenia, and asthenia.[25] A phase I/Ib study found that *KRAS*-mutant patients receiving trametinib and docetaxel had a 24% ORR, whereas those in the trametinib and pemetrexed arms had a 17% ORR.[26]

The first-in-human, phase I study of small molecule AMG 510, which specifically and irreversibly inhibits KRAS G12C by locking it in its guanosine diphosphate-bound state, was presented with results from 22 patients with advanced *KRAS* G12C solid tumors. Six patients had NSCLC; 2 experienced partial response after 6 weeks, and 2 patients had stable disease. The median treatment duration was 9.7 weeks; treatment was well-tolerated.[27] Two grade 3 AEs, namely, anemia and diarrhea, were reported; 68% of AEs were grade 1.

Studies assessing *KRAS* co-mutations have demonstrated lower clinical response rates in *KRAS*-mutant lung adenocarcinomas with

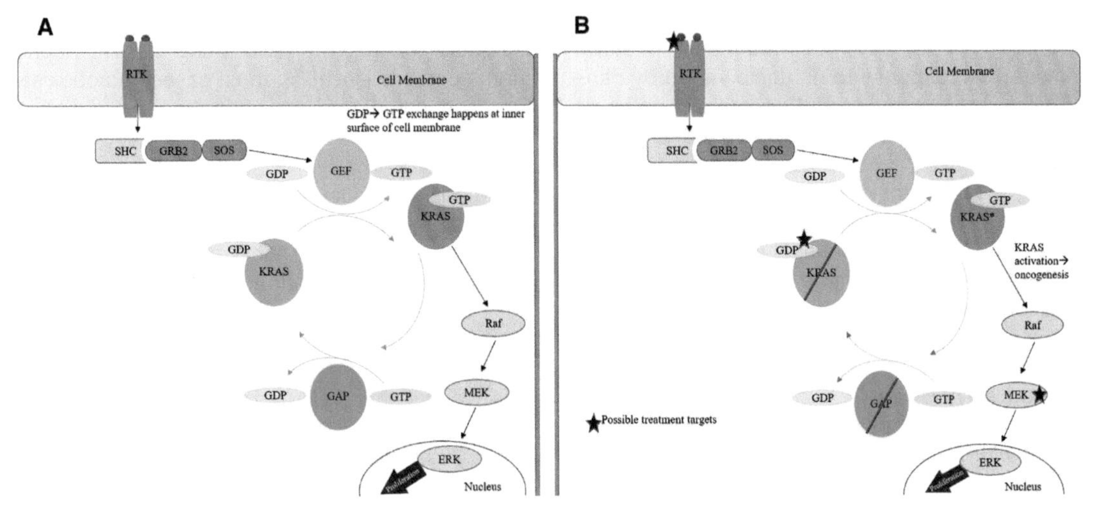

Fig. 1. (*A*) KRAS cycle in a KRAS wild-type cell—growth factors bind to receptor tyrosine kinases upstream of KRAS, which initiate signaling cascades via proteins with Src homology 2 (SH2). SH2 signaling domain proteins like growth factor receptor-bound protein 2 (GRB2) and Son of Sevenless (SOS) can then catalyze the KRAS guanosine diphosphate (GDP) → guanosine triphosphate (GTP) exchange via guanine nucleotide growth factor (GEF). GTP-bound KRAS can initiate signaling cascades like Raf/MEK/ERK. ERK can translocate into the nucleus activating a proliferative process. GTPase activating proteins (GAPs) mediate a GTP → GDP exchange resulting in inactivation of KRAS and homeostasis. (*B*) KRAS cycle in a mutant cell. The same upstream signaling pathways occurs in KRAS mutant cells. However, mutant KRAS is insensitive to GAPs, resulting in constitutive downstream action. * denotes possible treatment targets.

KEAP1 inactivation.[28] This subset of programmed death ligand 1 inhibitor–resistant tumors demonstrates lower programmed death ligand 1 expression and inactivation of the tumor suppressor *STK11/LKB1*, resulting in the accumulation of tumor-associated neutrophils with suppressive effects on T cells.[29] *LKB1* is mutated in approximately 30% of somatic lung adenocarcinomas.[30] A prior study showed NSCLC with *LKB1/KRAS* co-mutations responded distinctly to targeted therapies.[30] A murine study with *LKB1/KRAS* mutations or *p53/KRAS* mutations demonstrated a selective apoptotic response in *LKB1/KRAS*-mutated NSCLC tumors to the metformin-analog metabolic drug phenformin. Apoptosis was observed in NSCLC cell lines with mutated *LKB1* but not with *KRAS* WT.[31] *KRAS*-mutated lung cancer is a rapidly evolving area of research in the search for providing more treatment options for these patients with unmet need.

HUMAN EPIDERMAL GROWTH FACTOR RECEPTOR 2

Human epidermal growth factor receptor 2 (HER2), an erbB receptor tyrosine kinase family member, activates signaling through the PI3K–AKT and MEK–ERK pathways. HER2 is activated by homodimerization and heterodimerization with other members of the erbB family but does not have a known ligand.[32] HER2 overexpression is observed in 13% to 20% of lung cancer cases and is more common in women, never smokers, and lung adenocarcinomas.[33] *HER2* mutations are oncogenic and result in constitutive HER2 phosphorylation and activation and EGFR pathway stimulation.[34] *HER2* amplification and mutations are uncommon, representing 9% and 2% to 3% of cases, respectively.[35] *HER2* mutations occur in exons 18 to 21, usually in exon 20 at codon 776 with a 12 base pair duplication/insertion of the YVMA amino acid sequence. It is unclear if *HER2*-mutated tumors lead to worse patient outcomes compared with other variants.

A prospective study of the pan-HER TKI dacomitinib, which irreversibly binds HER2, HER1 (EGFR), and HER4, enrolled 30 patients with *HER2*-mutated (n = 26) or *HER2*-amplified (n = 4) NSCLC.[36] The ORR was 12% for patients with *HER2* mutation; no patients with amplification experienced tumor response. The median PFS was 3 months for all patients. In the *HER2*-mutant cohort, the median PFS was also 3 months with a 1-year survival rate of 44%. The pan-HER TKI, afatinib, showed limited results for *HER2*-mutated lung cancer. A single-arm phase II trial demonstrated a 12-week PFS of 53.8% and a medial PFS of 15.9 weeks with afatinib.[37] The median OS was 56 weeks.

Other small molecule TKIs have been investigated. The median PFS for neratinib alone, an irreversible pan-HER inhibitor,[38] was 2.9 months. The median PFS increased to 4 months with combined neratinib and temsirolimus treatment. A study showed that response to neratinib varied by cancer type, co-mutations, and concurrent pathway activation.[39] Patients with *HER2*-altered lung cancer (n = 26) had a low response rate, with 1 patient achieving an objective tumor response. For patients with *HER2*-mutated disease, although not limited to lung cancer, patients who did not show clinical benefit were more likely to have co-mutations in *TP53* and *HER3*. RAS/RAF pathway activation and coincident cell cycle checkpoint aberrations were associated with worse outcomes and no clinical benefit.

Antibody-based drugs have showed efficacy against *HER2*-mutated NSCLC. In a phase II trial, 18 patients with *HER2*-mutant lung adenocarcinomas were treated with T-DM1, demonstrating a 44% partial response rate and a 5-month median PFS.[40]

A retrospective study across European centers evaluated 101 patients with NSCLC with *HER2* mutations treated with chemotherapy and/or HER2-targeted therapy.[41] The median OS was 24 months for all patients, regardless of whether HER2-directed therapy was received. The ORR was highest for patients who received trastuzumab with or without chemotherapy or those who received T-DM1 at 50.9% with PFS 4.8 months.

The appropriate biomarker for selection remains elusive in this group of patients. At this time, mutation is the most predictive of response to HER2-directed therapy. Molecular aberrations in *HER2*-mutated lung cancers are heterogeneous, highlighted by varied effectiveness of HER2 kinase inhibitors. Important characteristics to consider are the type of mutation and the presence and degree of *HER2* amplification, expression, and concurrent pathway activation.

RET PROTO-ONCOGENE

RET is an receptor tyrosine kinase that mediates neural crest development; its activation causes cellular proliferation, migration, and differentiation.[42] *RET* gene alterations are most common in thyroid and lung cancers. Activating *RET* rearrangements preserve the tyrosine kinase domain of the 3′ *RET* gene and have various upstream 5′ fusion partners.[43] The most common fusion partner in NSCLC is *KIF5B*. *RET* fusions result in ligand-independent dimerization and downstream growth pathway activation.

RET fusions occur in approximately 1.4% of NSCLCs and 1.7% of adenocarcinomas[42] and are present mostly in patients 60 years or older with adenocarcinoma and no smoking history. A study of more than 4800 patients with varied malignancies undergoing NGS found that *RET* gene status occurred in 1.8%; most cases had coexisting, actionable genomic alterations, suggesting that successful treatment would involve custom combination approaches.[44]

Various multikinase TKIs have been tested on *RET*-rearranged NSCLC. A prospective phase II trial evaluating cabozantinib in 25 patients with *RET*-rearranged lung adenocarcinoma revealed a 28% ORR with a median PFS of 5.5 months and median OS of 9.9 months.[45] A phase II study investigating vandetanib in 19 *RET* fusion-positive patients found a 53% ORR and a 4.7-month median PFS.[46] A global, multicenter registry described treatment of 165 patients with *RET*-rearranged NSCLC, of which 53 had been treated with at least 1 RET inhibitor.[47] Cabozantinib, sunitinib, and vandetanib had ORRs of 37%, 22%, and 18%, respectively, and lenvatinib and nintedanib also caused tumor responses. In all patients, the median PFS was 2.3 months and the median OS was 6.8 months. Although these trials suggest inhibitory activity in *RET*-rearranged NSCLC, response to these multitargeted TKIs is modest and short lived.

RET-specific inhibitors are being evaluated to hopefully overcome the limitations of multikinase inhibitors. A report in patients with *RET*-altered malignancies showed that the potent RET inhibitor, LOXO-292, resulted in an ORR of 65% in 26 *RET*-altered patients with NSCLC. BLU-667, another selective RET inhibitor, demonstrated preclinical activity and clinical responses in patients with *RET*-altered NSCLC.[48] The study demonstrated an ORR of 58% for all patients (n = 48). BLU-667 was effective in patients with various *RET* fusion partners and against intracranial metastases.

MESENCHYMAL-EPITHELIAL TRANSITION

Mesenchymal-epithelial transition (*MET*) is a proto-oncogene that encodes for the transmembrane MET TKI. The binding of its ligand, hepatocyte growth factor, activates signaling pathways such as PI3K/AKT, MAPK, nuclear factor kappa B, and signal transducer and activator of transcription proteins, which promotes cell proliferation and invasion, blocking apoptosis, and increasing cell motility.[49–52] MET alterations are found in many cancers, including lung cancers, and induce tumor growth via protein overexpression and phosphorylation, gene amplification, rearrangement, and mutations.[52]

Protein overexpression and phosphorylation are the most common forms of MET-positive

NSCLC, whereas *MET* amplification is relatively rare and observed in approximately 2.2% of newly diagnosed adenocarcinoma and up to 7% of NSCLC cases.[53,54] Increased *MET* gene copy number is a negative prognosis factor in surgically resected NSCLC, with OS of 25.5 versus 47.5 months for patients with MET of 5 or more copies per cell and MET of less than 5 copies per cell, respectively.[54] Although the *KIF5B-MET* fusion has been reported in lung adenocarcinoma,[55] *MET* rearrangements are rare.

MET exon 14 alterations (4% of lung adenocarcinomas[53]) are diverse and drive tumorigenesis. They are associated with older age and significant smoking history.[56] Base substitutions or indels (usually deletions) in *MET* that disrupt the 3′ splice site or branch point of intron 13, or the 5′ splice site of intron 14, can lead to *MET* exon 14 skipping. Exon 14 skipping causes decreased MET ubiquitination by E3 ubiquitin-protein ligase CBL and MET degradation, leading to increased MET levels and downstream signaling, producing oncogenesis.[57] *MET* exon 14 alterations vary widely. A study found 126 different variants in 223 distinct exon 14 aberrations.[58]

Multitargeted TKIs have been used against MET in lung cancer, as have TKIs with increased MET sensitivity. In addition, monoclonal antibodies are being investigated in patients with MET-driven tumors. The dual MET/ALK inhibitor crizotinib showed antitumor responses in *MET* amplified and *MET* exon 14 mutated NSCLC.[58,59] In addition, crizotinib and cabozantinib have demonstrated antitumor response in patients with exon 14-altered lung adenocarcinoma.[60] A phase I study found that patients with high levels of *MET* amplification (MET/CEP7 $\geq$ 4) demonstrated antitumor activity with crizotinib, with median PFS of 6.7 months.[61]

Other studies have examined highly specific MET inhibitors for *MET* exon 14 mutated NSCLC. A phase II study investigated tepotinib for patients with NSCLC with *MET* exon 14 skipping mutations.[62] For patients with the variant detected with liquid biopsy, preliminary results demonstrated an ORR of 50.0% and a median PFS of 9.5 months. For patients with the variant detected by tissue biopsy, preliminary results demonstrated an ORR of 45.1% and a median PFS of 10.8 months.

Another phase II study investigated MET-specific inhibitor capmatinib in advanced NSCLC with *MET* exon 14 skipping mutations. Preliminary data from this study reported an ORR of 40.6% and a PFS of 5.42 months.[63] Patients without prior therapies had an ORR of 67.9% and a PFS of 9.69 months. Capmatinib also demonstrated a response against intracranial metastases, and patients tolerated the drug well.

It has been reported that *MET* amplification can increase to 5% to 22% after treatment with EGFR TKI therapy (erlotinib, gefitinib, osimertinib),[64,65] *MET* amplification is an alternative mechanism of resistance to EGFR TKIs in patients with EGFR mutation positive NSCLC.[66] Multiple combinations of MET and EGFR therapies are being evaluated in patients with resistant *EGFR* mutant NSCLC.

NEUREGULIN 1

Neuregulin 1 (*NRG1*) codes for the neuregulin protein.[67] In contrast to other NSCLC fusions, *NRG1* codes for a HER3 and HER4 tyrosine kinase receptor ligand. In these fusions, *NRG1* is the 3′ partner; other genes such as *CD74*, *RBPMS*, *WRN*, and *SDC4* are the 5′ partners.[68] The EGF domain of NRG1, located in the carboxy-terminal region and essential for receptor interaction, is preserved. *NRG1* fusions in lung cancer samples are found without other known driver mutations,[69] and *CD74-NRG1* fusions represent 1.7% of lung adenocarcinomas and occur most commonly in invasive mucinous adenocarcinoma,[70] an NSCLC subtype that represents 2% to 10% of all lung adenocarcinoma cases. This fusion causes PI3K-AKT pathway activation, which induces tumorigenesis.

Although there are few data available, an in vitro study showed that lapatinib and afatinib suppressed HER2, HER3, and ERK phosphorylation produced by *CD74-NERG1* fusions.[71] Two cases of patients with *NRG1* fusions showed response to afatinib, a HER2 inhibitor.[72] A *SLC3A2-NRG1* and a *CD74-NRG1* fusion demonstrated 12 months and 10 months PFS, respectively. In addition, a recent study reported a patient's *CD74-NRG1* fusion-positive NSCLC responded for 19 months to an investigational anti-HER3 monoclonal antibody.[73]

SUMMARY

Lung cancer represents a heterogenous group of thoracic tumors with distinct biologic and genomic characteristics. Clinical studies and molecular genotyping delineate appropriate therapy for many patients with NSCLC that represent precision treatment for the defined alteration. The list of genomic alterations is growing and broad molecular profiling for patients with advanced NSCLC is essential. Molecular selection defines specific populations that derive enhanced benefit from targeted treatment, and provide insights into potential mechanisms of resistance. Despite the progress that has been made, work is necessary to untangle the complex causes for primary and secondary resistance to therapy to make a dramatic impact on survival. Furthermore, interactions within the tumor microenvironment and with immune cells is becoming increasingly important, leading to exploration of combination therapies.

ACKNOWLEDGEMENTS

The author would like to thank Terrence C. Tsou, BS, of City of Hope Comprehensive Cancer Center (Duarte, CA, USA) and Haley C. Allen of Rice University (Houston, TX, USA) for their invaluable manuscript help.

DISCLOSURE

TT and HA have nothing to disclose.

KR- Consultant; Honoraria to myself, AstraZeneca, Boehringer Ingelheim, Calithera, Guardant, Precision Health. DSMC/Consultant; Honoraria to myself, Genentech, Tesaro

Grant/research support to institution (City of Hope): AbbVie, Acea, Adaptimmune, Boehringer Ingelheim, Bristol Myers Squibb, Genentech, GlaxoSmithKline, Guardant, Janssen, Loxo Oncology, Molecular Partners, Seattle Genetics, Spectrum, Takeda, Xcovery, Zeno.

REFERENCES

1. Govindan R, Ding L, Griffith M, et al. Genomic landscape of non-small cell lung cancer in smokers and never-smokers. Cell 2012;150(6):1121–34.
2. Samet JM, Avila-Tang E, Boffetta P, et al. Lung cancer in never smokers: clinical epidemiology and environmental risk factors. Clin Cancer Res 2009; 15(18):5626–45.
3. Kris MG, Johnson BE, Berry LD, et al. Using multiplexed assays of oncogenic drivers in lung cancers to select targeted drugs. JAMA 2014;311(19): 1998–2006.
4. Cardarella S, Ogino A, Nishino M, et al. Clinical, pathologic, and biologic features associated with BRAF mutations in non-small cell lung cancer. Clin Cancer Res 2013;19(16):4532–40.
5. Davies H, Bignell GR, Cox C, et al. Mutations of the BRAF gene in human cancer. Nature 2002; 417(6892):949–54.
6. Litvak AM, Paik PK, Woo KM, et al. Clinical characteristics and course of 63 patients with BRAF mutant lung cancers. J Thorac Oncol 2014;9(11):1669–74.
7. Paik PK, Arcila ME, Fara M, et al. Clinical characteristics of patients with lung adenocarcinomas harboring BRAF mutations. J Clin Oncol 2011; 29(15):2046–51.
8. Gautschi O, Pauli C, Strobel K, et al. A patient with BRAF V600E lung adenocarcinoma responding to vemurafenib. J Thorac Oncol 2012;7(10): e23–4.
9. Hyman DM, Puzanov I, Subbiah V, et al. Vemurafenib in multiple Nonmelanoma cancers with BRAF V600 mutations. N Engl J Med 2015;373(8):726–36.
10. Planchard D, Kim TM, Mazieres J, et al. Dabrafenib in patients with BRAF(V600E)-positive advanced non-small-cell lung cancer: a single-arm, multicentre, open-label, phase 2 trial. Lancet Oncol 2016;17(5):642–50.
11. Nakagawara A. Trk receptor tyrosine kinases: a bridge between cancer and neural development. Cancer Lett 2001;169(2):107–14.
12. Vaishnavi A, Le AT, Doebele RC. TRKing down an old oncogene in a new era of targeted therapy. Cancer Discov 2015;5(1):25–34.
13. Vaishnavi A, Capelletti M, Le AT, et al. Oncogenic and drug-sensitive NTRK1 rearrangements in lung cancer. Nat Med 2013;19(11):1469–72.
14. Farago AF, Taylor MS, Doebele RC, et al. Clinicopathologic features of non-small cell lung cancer (NSCLC) harboring an NTRK gene fusion. J Clin Oncol 2017;35(15_suppl):11580.
15. Doebele RC, Davis LE, Vaishnavi A, et al. An oncogenic NTRK fusion in a patient with soft-tissue sarcoma with response to the Tropomyosin-Related Kinase Inhibitor LOXO-101. Cancer Discov 2015; 5(10):1049–57.
16. Drilon A, Laetsch TW, Kummar S, et al. Efficacy of Larotrectinib in TRK fusion-positive cancers in adults and children. N Engl J Med 2018;378(8):731–9.
17. Farago AF, Le LP, Zheng Z, et al. Durable clinical response to Entrectinib in NTRK1-rearranged non-small cell lung cancer. J Thorac Oncol 2015; 10(12):1670–4.
18. Siena S, Doebele RC, Shaw AT, et al. Efficacy of entrectinib in patients (pts) with solid tumors and central nervous system (CNS) metastases: integrated analysis from three clinical trials. J Clin Oncol 2019;37(15_suppl):3017.
19. Prior IA, Lewis PD, Mattos C. A comprehensive survey of Ras mutations in cancer. Cancer Res 2012; 72(10):2457–67.
20. Dogan S, Shen R, Ang DC, et al. Molecular epidemiology of EGFR and KRAS mutations in 3,026 lung adenocarcinomas: higher susceptibility of women to smoking-related KRAS-mutant cancers. Clin Cancer Res 2012;18(22):6169–77.
21. Johnson ML, Sima CS, Chaft J, et al. Association of KRAS and EGFR mutations with survival in patients with advanced lung adenocarcinomas. Cancer 2013;119(2):356–62.
22. Campbell SL, Khosravi-Far R, Rossman KL, et al. Increasing complexity of Ras signaling. Oncogene 1998;17(11 Reviews):1395–413.

23. Ostrem JM, Peters U, Sos ML, et al. K-Ras(G12C) inhibitors allosterically control GTP affinity and effector interactions. Nature 2013;503:548.
24. Kohl NE, Omer CA, Conner MW, et al. Inhibition of farnesyltransferase induces regression of mammary and salivary carcinomas in ras transgenic mice. Nat Med 1995;1(8):792–7.
25. Jänne P, Shaw A, Pereira J, et al. Selumetinib plus docetaxel for KRAS-mutant advanced non-small-cell lung cancer: a randomised, multicentre, placebo-controlled, phase 2 study. Lancet Oncol 2013;14(1):38–47.
26. Gandara DR, Leighl N, Delord J-P, et al. A Phase 1/1b study evaluating trametinib plus docetaxel or pemetrexed in patients with advanced non–small cell lung cancer. J Thorac Oncol 2017;12(3):556–66.
27. Fakih M, O'Neil B, Price TJ, et al. Phase 1 study evaluating the safety, tolerability, pharmacokinetics (PK), and efficacy of AMG 510, a novel small molecule KRASG12C inhibitor, in advanced solid tumors. J Clin Oncol 2019;37(15_suppl):abst 3003.
28. Jeanson A, Tomasini P, Souquet-Bressand M, et al. Efficacy of immune checkpoint inhibitors in KRAS-mutant Non-Small Cell Lung Cancer (NSCLC). J Thorac Oncol 2019;14(6):1095–101.
29. Skoulidis F, Goldberg ME, Greenawalt DM, et al. STK11/LKB1 mutations and PD-1 inhibitor resistance in KRAS-mutant lung adenocarcinoma. Cancer Discov 2018;8(7):822–35.
30. Mahoney CL, Choudhury B, Davies H, et al. LKB1/KRAS mutant lung cancers constitute a genetic subset of NSCLC with increased sensitivity to MAPK and mTOR signalling inhibition. Br J Cancer 2009;100:370.
31. Shackelford David B, Abt E, Gerken L, et al. LKB1 inactivation dictates therapeutic response of non-small cell lung cancer to the metabolism drug phenformin. Cancer Cell 2013;23(2):143–58.
32. Peters S, Zimmermann S. Targeted therapy in NSCLC driven by HER2 insertions. Transl Lung Cancer Res 2014;3(2):84–8.
33. Mazieres J, Peters S, Lepage B, et al. Lung cancer that harbors an HER2 mutation: epidemiologic characteristics and therapeutic perspectives. J Clin Oncol 2013;31(16):1997–2003.
34. Wang SE, Narasanna A, Perez-Torres M, et al. HER2 kinase domain mutation results in constitutive phosphorylation and activation of HER2 and EGFR and resistance to EGFR tyrosine kinase inhibitors. Cancer Cell 2006;10(1):25–38.
35. Landi L, Cappuzzo F. HER2 and lung cancer. Expert Rev Anticancer Ther 2013;13(10):1219–28.
36. Kris MG, Camidge DR, Giaccone G, et al. Targeting HER2 aberrations as actionable drivers in lung cancers: phase II trial of the pan-HER tyrosine kinase inhibitor dacomitinib in patients with HER2-mutant or amplified tumors. Ann Oncol 2015;26(7):1421–7.
37. Dziadziuszko R, Smit EF, Dafni U, et al. Afatinib in NSCLC With HER2 mutations: results of the prospective, open-label phase II NICHE trial of European Thoracic Oncology Platform (ETOP). J Thorac Oncol 2019;14(6):1086–94.
38. Gandhi L, Bahleda R, Tolaney SM, et al. Phase I study of neratinib in combination with temsirolimus in patients with human epidermal growth factor receptor 2-dependent and other solid tumors. J Clin Oncol 2014;32(2):68–75.
39. Hyman DM, Piha-Paul SA, Won H, et al. HER kinase inhibition in patients with HER2- and HER3-mutant cancers. Nature 2018;554(7691):189–94.
40. Li BT, Shen R, Buonocore D, et al. Ado-Trastuzumab Emtansine for patients with HER2-mutant lung cancers: results from a phase II basket trial. J Clin Oncol 2018;36(24):2532–7.
41. Mazieres J, Barlesi F, Filleron T, et al. Lung cancer patients with HER2 mutations treated with chemotherapy and HER2-targeted drugs: results from the European EUHER2 cohort. Ann Oncol 2016;27(2):281–6.
42. Wang R, Hu H, Pan Y, et al. RET fusions define a unique molecular and clinicopathologic subtype of non-small-cell lung cancer. J Clin Oncol 2012;30(35):4352–9.
43. Drilon A, Hu ZI, Lai GGY, et al. Targeting RET-driven cancers: lessons from evolving preclinical and clinical landscapes. Nat Rev Clin Oncol 2018;15(3):151–67.
44. Kato S, Subbiah V, Marchlik E, et al. RET aberrations in diverse cancers: next-generation sequencing of 4,871 patients. Clin Cancer Res 2017;23(8):1988–97.
45. Drilon A, Rekhtman N, Arcila M, et al. Cabozantinib in patients with advanced RET-rearranged non-small-cell lung cancer: an open-label, single-centre, phase 2, single-arm trial. Lancet Oncol 2016;17(12):1653–60.
46. Yoh K, Seto T, Satouchi M, et al. Vandetanib in patients with previously treated RET-rearranged advanced non-small-cell lung cancer (LURET): an open-label, multicentre phase 2 trial. Lancet Respir Med 2017;5(1):42–50.
47. Gautschi O, Milia J, Filleron T, et al. Targeting RET in patients with RET-rearranged lung cancers: results from the global, multicenter RET registry. J Clin Oncol 2017;35(13):1403–10.
48. Gainor JF, Lee DH, Curigliano G, et al. Clinical activity and tolerability of BLU-667, a highly potent and selective RET inhibitor, in patients (pts) with advanced RET-fusion+ non-small cell lung cancer (NSCLC). J Clin Oncol 2019;37(15_suppl):abstr9008.

49. Bottaro DP, Rubin JS, Faletto DL, et al. Identification of the hepatocyte growth factor receptor as the c-met proto-oncogene product. Science 1991; 251(4995):802–4.
50. Cooper CS, Park M, Blair DG, et al. Molecular cloning of a new transforming gene from a chemically transformed human cell line. Nature 1984; 311(5981):29–33.
51. Ponzetto C, Bardelli A, Zhen Z, et al. A multifunctional docking site mediates signaling and transformation by the hepatocyte growth factor/scatter factor receptor family. Cell 1994;77(2): 261–71.
52. Sadiq AA, Salgia R. MET as a possible target for non-small-cell lung cancer. J Clin Oncol 2013; 31(8):1089–96.
53. Cancer Genome Atlas Research Network. Comprehensive molecular profiling of lung adenocarcinoma. Nature 2014;511(7511):543–50.
54. Cappuzzo F, Marchetti A, Skokan M, et al. Increased MET gene copy number negatively affects survival of surgically resected non-small-cell lung cancer patients. J Clin Oncol 2009;27(10):1667–74.
55. Stransky N, Cerami E, Schalm S, et al. The landscape of kinase fusions in cancer. Nat Commun 2014;5:4846.
56. Awad MM, Oxnard GR, Jackman DM, et al. MET Exon 14 mutations in non-small-cell lung cancer are associated with advanced age and stage-dependent MET genomic amplification and c-Met overexpression. J Clin Oncol 2016;34(7):721–30.
57. Drilon A. MET exon 14 alterations in lung cancer: exon skipping extends half-life. Clin Cancer Res 2016;22(12):2832–4.
58. Frampton GM, Ali SM, Rosenzweig M, et al. Activation of MET via diverse exon 14 splicing alterations occurs in multiple tumor types and confers clinical sensitivity to MET inhibitors. Cancer Discov 2015; 5(8):850–9.
59. Mendenhall MA, Goldman JW. MET-mutated NSCLC with major response to Crizotinib. J Thorac Oncol 2015;10(5):e33–4.
60. Paik PK, Drilon A, Fan PD, et al. Response to MET inhibitors in patients with stage IV lung adenocarcinomas harboring MET mutations causing exon 14 skipping. Cancer Discov 2015;5(8):842–9.
61. Camidge DR, Otterson GA, Clark JW, et al. Crizotinib in patients (pts) with MET-amplified non-small cell lung cancer (NSCLC): updated safety and efficacy findings from a phase 1 trial. J Clin Oncol 2018;36(15_suppl):9062.
62. Paik PK, Veillon R, Cortot AB, et al. Phase II study of tepotinib in NSCLC patients with METex14 mutations. J Clin Oncol 2019;37(15_suppl):9005.
63. Wolf J, Seto T, Han JY, et al. Capmatinib (INC280) in METΔex14-mutated advanced non-small cell lung cancer (NSCLC): efficacy data from the phase II GEOMETRY mono-1 study. J Clin Oncol 2019;37(15_suppl):abstr 9004.
64. Bean J, Brennan C, Shih JY, et al. MET amplification occurs with or without T790M mutations in EGFR mutant lung tumors with acquired resistance to gefitinib or erlotinib. Proc Natl Acad Sci U S A 2007; 104(52):20932–7.
65. Piotrowska Z, Thress KS, Mooradian M, et al. MET amplification (amp) as a resistance mechanism to osimertinib. J Clin Oncol 2017;35(15_suppl):9020.
66. Engelman JA, Zejnullahu K, Mitsudomi T, et al. MET amplification leads to gefitinib resistance in lung cancer by activating ERBB3 signaling. Science 2007;316(5827):1039–43.
67. McCoach CE, Doebele RC. The minority report: targeting the rare oncogenes in NSCLC. Curr Treat Options Oncol 2014;15(4):644–57.
68. Dhanasekaran SM, Balbin OA, Chen G, et al. Transcriptome meta-analysis of lung cancer reveals recurrent aberrations in NRG1 and Hippo pathway genes. Nat Commun 2014;5:5893.
69. Jonna S, Feldman RA, Swensen J, et al. Detection of NRG1 gene fusions in solid tumors. Clin Cancer Res 2019;25(16):4966–72.
70. Fernandez-Cuesta L, Plenker D, Osada H, et al. CD74-NRG1 fusions in lung adenocarcinoma. Cancer Discov 2014;4(4):415–22.
71. Nakaoku T, Tsuta K, Ichikawa H, et al. Druggable oncogene fusions in invasive mucinous lung adenocarcinoma. Clin Cancer Res 2014;20(12):3087–93.
72. Gay ND, Wang Y, Beadling C, et al. Durable response to Afatinib in lung adenocarcinoma harboring NRG1 gene fusions. J Thorac Oncol 2017;12(8):e107–10.
73. Drilon A, Somwar R, Mangatt BP, et al. Response to ERBB3-directed targeted therapy in NRG1-rearranged cancers. Cancer Discov 2018;8(6): 686–95.

Liquid Biopsies Using Circulating Tumor DNA in Non-Small Cell Lung Cancer

Bruna Pellini, MD[a], Jeffrey Szymanski, MD, PhD[b], Re-I. Chin, MD[b], Paul A. Jones, BS[b], Aadel A. Chaudhuri, MD, PhD[b,*]

KEYWORDS

- Circulating tumor DNA (ctDNA) • Non-small cell lung cancer (NSCLC) • Liquid biopsy
- Plasma genotyping

KEY POINTS

- A liquid biopsy is a test done on a body fluid sample (usually blood) to assess cancer.
- Circulating tumor DNA (ctDNA) can be measured by polymerase chain reaction (PCR) and next-generation sequencing (NGS)-based technologies.
- ctDNA testing is approved in clinical practice for recurrent or metastatic NSCLC when tissue testing is inadequate or not feasible.
- Major challenges of ctDNA technology include early-stage cancer detection and distinguishing tumor mutations from clonal hematopoiesis.

INTRODUCTION

The development of targeted therapies has substantially improved outcomes for a subset of patients with non-small cell lung cancer (NSCLC).[1] As treatments become more effective, they are also becoming more personalized, requiring novel testing strategies to identify driver mutations, track tumor evolution, and monitor disease recurrence.[2] Liquid biopsies offer a noninvasive way to monitor and personalize treatment for NSCLC.

A liquid biopsy refers to a clinical assay performed on a sample of bodily fluid for cancer assessment. For solid tumor malignancies, these assays typically assess either circulating tumor cells or cell-free circulating tumor DNA (ctDNA) in the blood.[3] In this article we will focus on ctDNA detection from blood plasma and clinical applications of this technology.[4,5]

CELL-FREE DNA

In both healthy and diseased individuals, nonencapsulated extracellular DNA fragments called cell-free DNA (cfDNA) are found in different bodily fluids.[10,11,12,13] Although the process is not well-studied, cfDNA is thought to be generated primarily through passive release from apoptotic and necrotic cells (**Fig. 1**).[6,7,14] As such, cfDNA fragments are usually 150 to 200 bp in length, roughly corresponding to the length of DNA wrapped around a single nucleosome.[15] cfDNA has a short half-life ranging between 16 minutes and 2.5 hours, making it an ideal substrate for studying tumor mutational dynamics as discussed later in this article.[16] In blood plasma, most cfDNA originates from nucleated peripheral blood cells and endothelial cells, and is present between ~1 and ~100 ng/mL.[17]

The amount of plasma cfDNA is dramatically increased in many disease states, often as a result

[a] Department of Medicine, Division of Oncology, Washington University School of Medicine, Division of Oncology Campus Box 8056, 660 South Euclid Avenue, St Louis, MO 63110, USA; [b] Department of Radiation Oncology, Division of Cancer Biology, Washington University School of Medicine, Radiation Oncology Campus Box 8224, 660 South Euclid Avenue, St Louis, MO 63110, USA
* Corresponding author.
E-mail address: aadel@wustl.edu

Thorac Surg Clin 30 (2020) 165–177
https://doi.org/10.1016/j.thorsurg.2020.01.005
1547-4127/20/

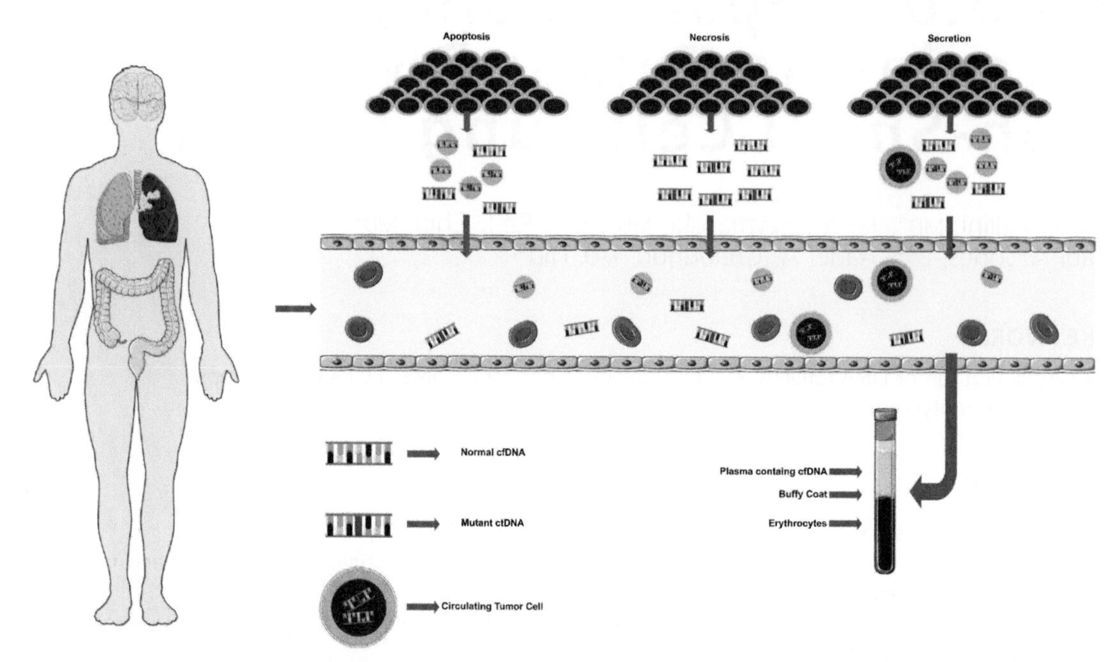

Fig. 1. Cell-free DNA generated by healthy endothelial cells and leukocytes, and ctDNA released from solid tumor malignant cells. Circulating tumor cells are also depicted.

of increased cell turnover.[2,3] In patients diagnosed with solid malignancies, DNA from cancer cells also contributes to plasma cfDNA and is referred to as ctDNA.[18] In lung cancer, ctDNA tends to be higher in patients with metastatic or locally advanced disease. Overall, ctDNA levels tend to increase with disease progression.[8]

CIRCULATING TUMOR DNA DETECTION METHODS

Methods used to detect DNA mutations in plasma are similar to those used on biopsied tissue, but tailored to meet some of the unique challenges of cfDNA as a substrate. Detection techniques can be broadly categorized by their scope of genomic coverage, from targeted allele-specific polymerase chain reaction (PCR) to next-generation sequencing (NGS) techniques such as hybrid capture NGS, whole exome sequencing and whole genome sequencing (**Table 1**). Common challenges for all detection methods include the low amount of ctDNA present in plasma, the abundant background of cfDNA arising from normal (nontumor) cells, and the uncertain origin of variants discovered.[8]

An additional challenge shared by all ctDNA assays is the potential for leukocyte genomic DNA contamination of samples.[48] Although some early ctDNA testing was performed on serum, where the total nucleic acid yield is higher, modern assays exclusively use plasma to avoid potential contamination from lysed blood cells.[20] To further prevent leukocyte genomic DNA in plasma samples, the College of American Pathologists and the American Society of Clinical Oncology now recommend separating plasma from blood cells within 6 hours of collection in EDTA tubes, and the International Association for the Study of Lung Cancer recommends processing blood within 2 hours.[21] Alternatively, leukocyte stabilization tubes allow specimens to sit for up to 48 hours before processing.[22] No standard collection volume has been established for ctDNA assays. However, to increase analytical sensitivity, plasma volumes of 10-mL or higher are common, requiring that multiple EDTA vacutainers be drawn per assay.[20]

Allele-Specific Polymerase Chain Reaction

PCR-based assays are typically used when detecting single mutations or small panels of well-characterized variants, to query for targeted therapeutic eligibility or evidence of acquired resistance.[16] Allele-specific PCR (AS-PCR, also known as amplification refractory mutation system) can report allele frequencies for single nucleotide variants in plasma cfDNA.[16] In conventional PCR, primers are designed to anneal outside of the sequence region of interest, while in AS-PCR, 3′ primers overlap the region of interest. AS-PCR primers uniquely complementary to either variant-containing or wild-type sequences are

Table 1
Comparison of Techniques Used for ctDNA Detection

Technique	Example Technologies	Scale of Analysis	Method	Detection Limit (as % of cfDNA)	Cost	Assay Personalization	Advantages	Limitations
AS-PCR	Cobas EGFR mutation test v2 (Roche)	Single-locus or multiplexed assays	Preferentially amplifies rare mutant DNA molecules	~0.1%–1%	$	Some required	Ease of use; ideal for detecting recurrent "hotspot" point mutations	Limited multiplexing ability; analytical sensitivity not as low as digital PCR
Digital PCR	Digital PCR ddPCR BEAMing	Single-locus or multiplexed assays	Partitions target DNA into different reactions for massively parallel quantitative PCR	~0.04%–0.1%	$$	Some required	High sensitivity	Limited multiplexing ability
WGS	WGS Plasma-Seq PARE	Genome wide	NGS of whole genome	~10%	$$–$$$	Not required	Entire genome is interrogated	Low sensitivity; mostly limited to SCNA detection; requires in-depth genomics and bioinformatics analysis

(*continued on next page*)

Table 1
(continued)

Technique	Example Technologies	Scale of Analysis	Method	Detection Limit (as % of cfDNA)	Cost	Assay Personalization	Advantages	Limitations
Retrotransposon-based Amplicon NGS	FAST-SeqS mFAST-SeqS WALDO	Genome-wide retrotransposon sites	PCR amplification of retrotransposon insertion sites before NGS analysis	~5%	$$	Not required	Rapid aneuploidy assessment with lower cost than WGS	Limited to aneuploidy detection
WES	WES	Exome wide	NGS of whole exome	~5%	$$$	Not required	Entire exome is interrogated	Typically low sensitivity; requires in-depth genomics and bioinformatics analysis
Multiplex PCR-based NGS	TAm-Seq Enhanced TAm-Seq Safe-SeqS Natera	Targeted sequencing	PCR amplification enriches targets before NGS analysis	~0.01%–2.0%	$$	Some required	High sensitivity (modern methods)	Less comprehensive than WGS or WES; requires bioinformatics analysis

Hybrid capture-based NGS	CAPP-Seq TEC-Seq Guardant360 FoundationOne Liquid	Targeted sequencing	Subset of exome is hybridized to biotinylated probes and captured for NGS analysis	~0.001%–0.5%	$$	Typically not required	High sensitivity; detects multiple mutation types; broadly applicable without personalization	Less comprehensive than WGS or WES; requires bioinformatics analysis
Combination approaches	CAPP-Seq + GRP CancerSEEK UroSEEK	Single locus to genome wide	Combines different ctDNA detection methods sometimes including protein biomarkers	Variable	$$–$$$	Variable	Improved detection compared with standard ctDNA analysis alone in certain settings	More time and resource intensive than individual approaches

Abbreviations: ARMS, amplification-refractory mutation system; BEAMing, beads, emulsion, amplification and magnetics; CAPP-Seq, cancer personalized profiling by deep sequencing; ctDNA, circulating tumor deoxyribonucleic acid; FAST-SeqS, fast aneuploidy screening test-sequencing system; GRP, genome representation profiling; mFAST-SeqS, modified FAST-SeqS; PARE, personalized analysis of rearranged ends; PASA, amplification of specific alleles; Plasma-Seq, plasma sequencing; Safe-SeqS, safe sequencing system; SCNA, somatic copy-number alternation; TAm-Seq, tagged amplicon deep sequencing; TEC-Seq, targeted error correction sequencing; WALDO, within sample aneuploidy detection; WES, whole exome sequencing; WGS, whole genome sequencing.

Adapted from Chin RI, Chen K, Usmani A, et al. Detection of solid tumor molecular residual disease (MRD) using circulating tumor DNA (ctDNA). Mol Diagnosis Ther. 2019;23(3):311–31; with permission.

used in separate reactions, and amplification occurs only when the template DNA perfectly matches the 3′ primer.[23] AS-PCR assays are an attractive option for rapid clinical testing, with a quantitative readout using standard real-time PCR equipment. The cobas epidermal growth factor receptor (EGFR) mutation test v2 (Roche, Basel, Switzerland) is an example of an AS-PCR assay that queries 42 different EGFR mutations.[24] Most clinical laboratories already perform real-time PCR assays, reagents are relatively inexpensive, and interpretation of the spectrophotometric signal is straightforward. Important drawbacks of AS-PCR include limited multiplexing and sensitivities in plasma of only about 70% to 80%.[12,25]

Droplet Digital Polymerase Chain Reaction

Digital droplet PCR (ddPCR) measures tens of thousands of PCR reactions in nanoliter-scale droplets, evaluating each reaction as a discrete measurement.[26] ddPCR has superior analytical sensitivity to AS-PCR, with a detection limit in the range of 0.04% to 0.10%.[12,54] However, currently the clinical benefits of increased sensitivity are unclear as ddPCR and AS-PCR performed similarly as confirmatory tests for patients positive for the EGFR T790M mutation in plasma.[28] Both PCR methods have a substantially faster turnaround time than NGS-based methods, with most results returned within 72 hours compared to 1 to 2 weeks for massively parallel sequencing.[29] Like AS-PCR, a drawback of ddPCR is the limited ability to multiplex the assay to query mutations in multiple genes simultaneously.[12]

Targeted Next-Generation Sequencing

As clinically useful molecular targets continue to accumulate, NGS becomes an increasingly important testing method in NSCLC. Although whole exome and even whole genome sequencing can potentially offer more comprehensive genomic information, most ctDNA NGS assays in clinical use are more targeted, using either hybrid capture panels or amplicon-based NGS.[30] Both of these methods, when applied to ctDNA detection, involve high-depth NGS to detect low allele frequency mutations in the plasma.[12]

Mutant allele frequency of ctDNA in plasma varies with cancer stage and treatment effect, typically being significantly lower in early-stage disease and after cytotoxic treatment. Reliably detecting ctDNA mutations in lung cancer patients with NGS, especially for post-treatment molecular residual disease (MRD) detection, requires extraordinary sensitivity.[8,22,32] This sensitivity can be achieved through personalized high depth sequencing, with raw nondeduplicated depths of 50,000× commonly achieved, along with digital error suppression techniques, enabling detection of variants with allele frequencies as low as approximately 10^{-4}.[8,9,32,33] However, bridge amplification sequencing has an error rate of approximately 10^{-3},[34] meaning that any rare variant discovered at this high depth is likely to originate from ex vivo sequencing errors than from a real, in vivo ctDNA mutation. To account for this, modern NGS-based techniques use barcoded sequencing adapters and bioinformatic error suppression to reduce this technical error rate significantly and enable ultra-low level ctDNA detection.[8,32,33]

CLINICAL USE OF LIQUID BIOPSIES

The College of American Pathologists, the International Association for the Study of Lung Cancer, and the Association for Molecular Pathology recommend molecular testing from tumor tissue in patients with NSCLC.[35] ctDNA testing should only be used when there is insufficient tissue for molecular testing or when tissue cannot be obtained.[35] Of note, liquid biopsies may spare patients from major complications associated with computed tomography-guided lung biopsy that occur in approximately 5% of patients.[21]

In clinical practice, ctDNA assessment from blood plasma is the mostly widely used liquid biopsy approach, with Zill and colleagues[36] recently reporting results from 21,807 patients with advanced cancer assessed using the Guardant360 assay (Guardant Health, Redwood City, CA). ctDNA analysis can identify actionable tumor mutations at the time of diagnosis and/or recurrence of patients with advanced/metastatic adenocarcinoma of the lung.[21] Additionally, ctDNA testing is recommended if a patient is diagnosed with squamous cell carcinoma and is a never smoker or young patient, or if a patient has a non-squamous component on tumor histology. In clinical practice, we can usually forego the need to perform tissue NGS if the ctDNA molecular test is positive for an actionable mutation.[21] This recommendation applies to patients being treated with targeted therapy and chemotherapy and/or immunotherapy.[12,21] In addition, different proof-of-concept studies have demonstrated ctDNA's ability to detect post-treatment MRD, which was shown to be prognostic.[12,22,32,37] Still, ctDNA analysis for MRD detection is not yet approved for clinical practice.

As an example of ctDNA's impact in clinical practice, PCR-based techniques are used to detect EGFR exon 19 deletions and L858R single nucleotide variants in plasma, reaching sensitivities as high as 100% (range, 78%–100%) while maintaining high specificity (93%–100%).[38] Detection of EGFR mutations are of extreme clinical importance because their detection changes the management of NSCLC patients. If an EGFR exon 19 deletion or L858R mutation is detected, patients should be treated with an EGFR tyrosine kinase inhibitor in the first-line setting rather than chemotherapy or immunotherapy.[39] Although PCR allows rapid detection of genetic alterations without extensive genomic analysis, thus translating to cost-effective techniques, it only enables monitoring of a limited number of known mutations. Conversely, NGS-based techniques can interrogate larger regions of multiple genes in a single run. Limitations of NGS-based technologies include longer processing and analysis time than PCR, and higher costs (see **Table 1**).[40]

As of 2019, the only test approved by the US Food and Drug Administration for the molecular analysis of liquid biopsy specimens in NSCLC is the cobas test (Roche), an AS-PCR assay that queries EGFR mutations.[24] Nevertheless, assay development and clinical implementation are outpacing regulatory approval. At leading cancer centers, ctDNA testing is being performed routinely in patients with solid malignancies using either in-house laboratory developed tests (ie, MSK-ACCESS[41]) or commercially available assays (ie, Inivata [Cambridge, UK][42] and Guardant Health[31,43]) that query panels of potentially actionable mutations, which may inform clinical decision-making.

Tumor Profiling at Diagnosis

Even though ctDNA testing is being used in clinical practice, it is not the gold standard for actionable mutation assessment in newly diagnosed metastatic NSCLC owing to concerns regarding sensitivity.[21] Sabari and colleagues[44] illustrated ctDNA sensitivity limitations in a prospective study with 210 patients with advanced NSCLC. The detection rate of known tumor-derived somatic mutations in patients receiving systemic therapy was only 42.9% when using a 21-gene hybrid capture NGS assay. Even though ctDNA analysis detected a variety of mutations with a shorter turnaround time, their findings support that negative plasma genotyping requires confirmatory tumor testing to rule out a false negative result.[44]

In an attempt to prove ctDNA noninferiority to physician discretion standard-of-care (SOC) tumor genotyping, Leighl and colleagues[34] conducted a prospective study (the NILE study), which enrolled 307 patients with newly diagnosed stage IIIB and stage IV NSCLC, and compared physician's choice tissue genotyping with plasma genotyping using the Guardant360 platform to detect somatic ctDNA mutations. The authors compared these tests' performances in identifying 8 guideline-recommended biomarkers (EGFR mutations, ALK fusions, ROS1 fusions, BRAF V600E mutation, RET fusions, MET amplifications, MET exon 14 skipping variants and ERBB2 [HER2] mutation), in addition to KRAS mutations. ctDNA testing identified significantly more patients (77.0% vs 27.3%) with a guideline-recommended biomarker than physician-discretion SOC genotyping (60.0% vs 21.3%). Overall clinical sensitivity of ctDNA relative to tissue was 80% for the detection of any guideline-recommended biomarker. When restricting analysis to the targets approved by the US Food and Drug Administration, namely actionable genomic alterations in EGFR, ALK, ROS1, and BRAF, ctDNA concordance with tissue testing was greater than 98.2% with 100% positive predictive value.[34] Also, although EGFR mutations and ALK fusions were tested in the majority of patients (83% and 80% of patients, respectively) by physician SOC tissue genotyping, the other guideline-recommended mutations were tested in only one-quarter to one-third of cases. Overall, ctDNA testing increased the detection of somatic mutations by 48%, including those with tissue that was not assessed or yielded insufficient or negative results.[34] Another advantage of ctDNA testing was a significantly shorter turnaround time of a median of 9 days compared to 15 days for tissue genotyping.

This study's results suggest that panel-based ctDNA testing is noninferior to physician-discretion SOC genotyping and has advantages including a shorter turnaround time, mutational assessment not reliant on a physician ordering each molecular test separately, and the potential to identify mutations missed by tissue genotyping.[34] Thus, in the future, clinicians may implement parallel plasma genotyping for newly diagnosed metastatic NSCLC to avoid incomplete genotyping and diagnostic delays.

Another study of tissue genotyping in patients diagnosed with advanced NSCLC (stages IIIB and IV) in the community setting noted that only 59% of the 814 patients met the guideline recommendations for EGFR and ALK testing and only 8% underwent comprehensive tissue genomic profiling.[45] Barriers to complete genomic profiling included lack of tissue for molecular analysis, and reliance on an oncologist's orders to have each genotyping test performed. ctDNA testing may thus improve rates of molecular testing in the community setting, enabling the identification of more patients who are candidates for targeted therapies.

Circulating Tumor DNA Testing for Targeted Therapy

All patients diagnosed with advanced/metastatic nonsquamous NSCLC and younger patients, nonsmokers or light smokers diagnosed with squamous NSCLC should be tested for EGFR mutations, ALK fusions, ROS1 fusions, BRAF V600E mutation, RET fusions, MET amplifications, MET exon 14 skipping variants, and ERBB2 (HER2) mutations according to different society guidelines (American Society of Clinical Oncology, National Comprehensive Cancer Network, International Association for the Study of Lung Cancer).[21,45,46] Molecular testing should be performed using tissue samples, however ctDNA testing can be performed if tumor tissue is inadequate or not obtainable in order to identify actionable mutations.[21]

Epidermal growth factor receptor mutations

In 2015, Mok and colleagues[25] published the results of a prospective study assessing the concordance rates between plasma and tissue genotyping for EGFR mutation in 238 patients diagnosed with NSCLC. The authors described a concordance rate of 88% between plasma and tissue, with a sensitivity of 75% and specificity of 96% for blood testing of EGFR mutations.[25] Additionally, dynamic changes in ctDNA EGFR mutational status correlated strongly with clinical outcomes. Patients who were ctDNA-positive for EGFR mutation at baseline that later became undetectable by cycle 3 had significantly longer progression-free and overall survival than patients with persistently detectable EGFR mutations.[25] These results suggest that EGFR ctDNA testing is both predictive and prognostic, and that dynamic changes in blood-based EGFR testing may be useful as a biomarker for treatment response.

Resistance to EGFR tyrosine kinase inhibitors is a well-described phenomenon.[2] Approximately 60% of patients treated with a first-line EGFR tyrosine kinase inhibitor (erlotinib, afatinib, gefitinib) who develop treatment resistance, acquire an EGFR T790M mutation.[47] In 2017, Jenkins and colleagues[48] assessed the cobas plasma test to detect T790M mutations from plasma cfDNA in patients enrolled onto the AURA extension and AURA2 studies. Their results revealed that T790M mutations were detected in plasma of only 61% of the patients whose tumor harbored such a mutation. Although other techniques such as ddPCR may have a higher sensitivity (71%)[38] to detect the T790M mutation, the discrepancy between plasma and tissue genotyping for this mutation may be more common than for exon 19 deletions or L858R variants.[38] As such, tissue-based testing is preferable whenever feasible to query EGFR T790M mutational status.[21,38,46,48]

Anaplastic lymphoma kinase (ALK) rearrangements

Although there are substantial data on EGFR plasma genotyping, data on ALK rearrangement assessment using ctDNA in treatment-naïve patients is more limited.[21] In the NILE study,[34] ctDNA sensitivity to detect ALK fusions in plasma was 62.5%.[34] This prospective cohort of 282 patients with ctDNA testing that included assessment of ALK rearrangements is the largest to date. Retrospective data suggest that quantitative PCR is a marginal method for the detection of ALK rearrangements in plasma.[21] Even though ddPCR is generally more sensitive than quantitative PCR at detecting mutations in cell-free DNA, a large prospective study using this technology has not been conducted for ALK fusions.[21]

Circulating Tumor DNA Testing for Immunotherapy

Immune checkpoint inhibitors (ICIs) have changed the treatment landscape for patients with NSCLC.[49] Recent studies suggest that high tumor mutational burden (TMB) is associated with clinical benefit from ICIs.[49] Nonetheless, 30% of patients with NSCLC do not have adequate tissue available for standard biomarker testing.[49] In this setting, Chaudhuri and colleagues[22] and Gandara and colleagues[49] reported on the development of novel assays to measure TMB from blood plasma ctDNA results. Gandara and colleagues[49] used samples from patients enrolled on the POPLAR[50] and OAK[51] studies to evaluate and validate their test, respectively, which was based on the FoundationOne hybrid capture NGS assay (Foundation Medicine Inc, Cambridge, MA). The authors found that TMB extrapolated from blood plasma correlated with tissue TMB. Also, when variant allele fractions were more than 1%, the concordance rate between tissue and blood TMB was very high ($r^2 = 0.998$).[49] Importantly, samples from patients enrolled on the POPLAR study demonstrated that a blood-derived TMB (bTMB) of 16 or greater was associated with improved progression-free survival (PFS) and overall survival (OS) with atezolizumab versus docetaxel, compared with the full biomarker-evaluable population.[49] When tested in the OAK study, there remained a significant PFS benefit for patients with a bTMB of 16 or greater treated with atezolizumab; however, the OS benefit compared to the general biomarker-evaluable population was not seen until a higher cutpoint of bTMB≥24.[49] Interestingly, a high bTMB did not significantly correlate with high tumor programmed death ligand 1 (PD-L1) expression; however, the authors showed that these factors independently contributed to the benefit of immunotherapy, with PFS outcomes being best in those with both high tumor PD-L1 and high bTMB.[49] These findings suggest that blood plasma-derived TMB is a potential noninvasive biomarker to predict benefit from ICIs.

Finally, Goldberg and colleagues[52] demonstrated a strong correlation between longitudinal ctDNA changes, radiographic response, OS, and PFS in patients with metastatic NSCLC treated with immune checkpoint inhibitors. Among 49 patients enrolled onto their study, 28 had somatic mutations that were identified in baseline plasma.[52] The study focused on these 28 patients, who had serial ctDNA analysis during ICI therapy which was compared with tumor size measured by computed tomography analyzed by RECIST 1.1.[53] ctDNA response was defined as more than a 50% decrease in mutant allele fraction from baseline followed by a second confirmatory measurement. Their results revealed that ctDNA response was seen more rapidly than radiographic response, occurring a median of 42.5 days earlier. Additionally, ctDNA response was associated with improved PFS and OS, with a hazard ratio of 0.29 and 0.17, respectively.[52] Although compelling, the small size of this study and the lack of independent validation of its results make it challenging to translate into clinical practice yet.

LIQUID BIOPSY CHALLENGES

ctDNA analysis is complicated by several factors including intertumoral and intratumoral heterogeneity, clonal hematopoiesis (CH) and the technical challenge of detecting variants at low allele fractions.[12,54,19] With the constant clonal selection that tumors undergo during different lines of treatment, single-site biopsies are unable to reflect the complexity of the entire tumor genomic landscape.[2] Patients may have intratumoral heterogeneity (variable genomic landscape within one site of disease), and intertumoral heterogeneity (molecular differences between the primary tumor and metastatic sites), which may reflect discordant genotyping results between plasma and tissue.[37,55–57] Furthermore, the sensitivity of ctDNA detection depends on ctDNA levels.[58,59] Patients diagnosed with advanced/metastatic NSCLC often possess 10% or higher levels of ctDNA, whereas individuals with localized disease typically harbor 1% or less ctDNA in their plasma.[12] As such, highly sensitive assays are necessary to detect ctDNA in patients, especially in those with earlier stages of disease.[22,32,37,58,27,60]

CH is another challenge facing ctDNA analysis.[48,61] CH arises when age-dependent acquired mutations accumulate in hematopoietic progenitor cells, leading to genetically distinct subpopulations that contribute disproportionately to the population of mature blood cells.[62,63] In the measurement of ctDNA, CH can result in false-positive results owing to detection of nonreference variants in the plasma,[64–67] some of which are in genes like TP53 and KRAS that are frequently mutated in solid tumors.[48,61] Although the prevalence of CH has previously been reported to be approximately 30% in adults over 60 years of age,[48] Swanton and associates[61] presented findings from the ongoing Circulating Cell-free Genome Atlas Study at the 2018 American Society of Clinical Oncology meeting showing that CH was detected in 92% of patients with a variant allele fraction of more than 0.1%. Because most of plasma cfDNA is composed of DNA arising from nucleated hematopoietic cells, CH-related mutations can thus lead to false-positive results. This issue was reported by Hu and colleagues[48] in a cohort of patients with advanced NSCLC. The authors performed paired genotyping of peripheral blood cells and plasma, and detected false-positive ctDNA genotyping for KRAS and TP53 mutations owing to CH.[48] With modern NGS-based assays that possess high sensitivity, there is thus a high likelihood of identifying CH, which can be misinterpreted as tumoral mutations.[12] Therefore, caution is advised when interpreting plasma genotyping results from commercial vendors, especially given that these assays do not filter variants present in matched peripheral blood leukocytes.[12,48,61]

Analytical aspects also pose a challenge to ctDNA analysis. Given the short half-life of ctDNA and the possibility of contamination of plasma cfDNA with DNA from healthy leukocytes, it is crucial that blood be collected in specialized tubes or be processed and stored quickly after collection. The isolation of cfDNA from plasma has yet to be completely standardized and multiple protocols and kits have been developed.[22,68] ctDNA fragments are often shorter than healthy cfDNA, and both are substantially smaller than genomic cellular DNA derived from blood leukocytes.[6,8,69,70] Thus, enriching for shorter cfDNA fragments may boost the sensitivity of ctDNA detection.[71] Given that ctDNA typically is a small fraction of total cfDNA, very sensitive methods to reliably detect mutant DNA molecules are required.[8,32] Finally, discordances have been reported between ctDNA assay platforms, which could be related to different sets of mutations queried among other factors including the analytical techniques used.[38,72] Further cross-validation and standardization between assays and tissue testing need to be rigorously performed if we are to expand the clinical utility of ctDNA testing in standard clinical practice.

FUTURE DIRECTIONS

ctDNA assays currently in clinical use are largely restricted to the diagnostic testing of recurrent and/or metastatic disease, to aid in the selection of targeted therapies when tissue is inadequate or unavailable.[21] However, as ctDNA assay sensitivity increases, new applications will emerge, including testing in lieu of tissue even when it is available, and potentially screening and MRD monitoring.[8] Better screening for lung cancers is especially important because the 5-year OS is approximately 70% at stage 1,[73] whereas the OS is only 16% at stage IV.[74] In addition, only 5% of patients receive annual low-dose computed tomography screening. So far, hybrid capture panels have shown insufficient sensitivity in small screening studies.[73] Nevertheless, higher sensitivity assays have shown promise for MRD detection in small clinical studies.[22,32,37] Optimizations to further lower the detection limit while maintaining specificity could potentially enable early cancer screening as well. We also envision that, with the expansion of mutational targets queried by ctDNA assays coupled with the proliferation of precision therapeutics, we can offer more patients molecularly targeted agents through umbrella clinical trials.[75]

SUMMARY

- A liquid biopsy is a clinical assay performed on a sample of body fluid to assess cancer.
- Liquid biopsy ctDNA assays commonly refer to the detection of tumor-specific mutations in the blood plasma of patients with cancer.
- ctDNA detection can be performed using ultra-sensitive PCR- and NGS-based techniques.
- ctDNA testing may not be sensitive enough to detect certain actionable mutations reliably like EGFR T790M.
- ctDNA testing should be used in clinical practice for recurrent or metastatic NSCLC only when tissue cannot be obtained or is insufficient for molecular analysis.
- ctDNA results may be confounded by CH, especially an issue for commercial assays where matched leukocytes are not sequenced.
- Further cross-validation between ctDNA assays and with tissue testing needs to be rigorously performed.
- Future directions include using ctDNA to molecularly guide umbrella trial enrollment, detect MRD, and potentially enable early cancer screening.

DISCLOSURE

A.A. Chaudhuri is a scientific advisor/consultant for Geneoscopy, Roche Sequencing Solutions and Tempus Labs; has received speaker honoraria and travel support from Varian Medical Systems, Roche Sequencing Solutions, and Foundation Medicine; receives research support from Roche Sequencing Solutions; and is an inventor of intellectual property licensed to Biocognitive Labs. The other authors have nothing to disclose.

REFERENCES

1. Herbst RS, Morgensztern D, Boshoff C. The biology and management of non-small cell lung cancer. Nature 2018. https://doi.org/10.1038/nature25183.
2. Pellini Ferreira B, Morgensztern D. Cell-free DNA in cancer diagnosis and follow-up. In: Govindan R, Devarakonda S, editors. Cancer genomics for the clinician. New York: Demos Medical Publishing; 2019. p. 115–26.
3. Diaz LA, Bardelli A. Liquid biopsies: genotyping circulating tumor DNA. J Clin Oncol 2014;32(6): 579–86.
4. Sacher AG, Komatsubara KM, Oxnard GR. Application of plasma genotyping technologies in non–small cell lung cancer: a practical review. J Thorac Oncol 2017;12(9):1344–56.
5. Rolfo C, Manca P, Salgado R, et al. Multidisciplinary molecular tumour board: a tool to improve clinical practice and selection accrual for clinical trials in patients with cancer. ESMO Open 2018;3(5):e000398.
6. Jahr S, Hentze H, Englisch S, et al. DNA fragments in the blood plasma of cancer patients: quantitations and evidence for their origin from apoptotic and necrotic cells. Cancer Res 2001;61(4):1659–65.
7. Choi JJ, Reich CF, Pisetsky DS. The role of macrophages in the in vitro generation of extracellular DNA from apoptotic and necrotic cells. Immunology 2005;115(1):55–62.
8. Chin RI, Chen K, Usmani A, et al. Detection of solid tumor molecular residual disease (MRD) using circulating tumor DNA (ctDNA). Mol Diagn Ther 2019;23(3):311–31.
9. Chaudhuri AA, Chabon JJ, Lovejoy AF, et al. Early detection of molecular residual disease in localized

lung cancer by circulating tumor DNA profiling. Cancer Discov 2017;7(12):1394–403.
10. Dudley JC, Schroers-Martin J, Lazzareschi DV, et al. Detection and surveillance of bladder cancer using urine tumor DNA. Cancer Discov 2018;10. https://doi.org/10.1158/2159-8290.CD-18-0825.
11. Springer SU, Chen C-H, Rodriguez Pena MDC, et al. Non-invasive detection of urothelial cancer through the analysis of driver gene mutations and aneuploidy. Elife 2018;7:1–27.
12. De Mattos-Arruda L, Mayor R, Ng CKY, et al. Cerebrospinal fluid-derived circulating tumour DNA better represents the genomic alterations of brain tumours than plasma. Nat Commun 2015;6:1–6.
13. Husain H, Nykin D, Bui N, et al. Cell-free DNA from ascites and pleural effusions: molecular insights into genomic aberrations and disease biology. Mol Cancer Ther 2017;16:948–55.
14. Chaudhuri AA, Binkley MS, Osmundson EC, et al. Predicting radiotherapy responses and treatment outcomes through analysis of circulating tumor DNA. Semin Radiat Oncol 2015;25(4):305–12.
15. Corcoran RB, Chabner BA. Application of cell-free DNA analysis to cancer treatment. N Engl J Med 2018;379:1754–65.
16. Yao W, Mei C, Nan X, et al. Evaluation and comparison of in vitro degradation kinetics of DNA in serum, urine and saliva: a qualitative study. Gene 2016;590: 142–1488.
17. Alborelli I, Generali D, Jermann P, et al. Cell-free DNA analysis in healthy individuals by next-generation sequencing: a proof of concept and technical validation study. Cell Death Dis 2019;10: 534.
18. Stroun M, Anker P, Lyautey J, et al. Isolation and characterization of DNA from the plasma of cancer patients. Eur J Cancer Clin Oncol 1987;23(6): 707–12.
19. Hu Y, Ulrich BC, Supplee J, et al. False-positive plasma genotyping due to clonal hematopoiesis. Clin Cancer Res 2018;24(18):4437–43.
20. El Messaoudi S, Rolet F, Mouliere F, et al. Circulating cell free DNA: preanalytical considerations. Clin Chim Acta 2013. https://doi.org/10.1016/j.cca.2013.05.022.
21. Rolfo C, Mack PC, Scagliotti GV, et al. Liquid biopsy for advanced non-small cell lung cancer (NSCLC): a statement paper from the IASLC. J Thorac Oncol 2018. https://doi.org/10.1016/j.jtho.2018.05.030.
22. Parpart-Li S, Bartlett B, Popoli M, et al. The effect of preservative and temperature on the analysis of circulating tumor DNA. Clin Cancer Res 2017; 23(10):2471–7.
23. Newton CR, Graham A, Heptinstall LE, et al. Analysis of any point mutation in DNA. The amplification refractory mutation system (ARMS). Nucleic Acids Res 1989;17(7):2503–16.
24. Malapelle U, Sirera R, Jantus-Lewintre E, et al. Profile of the Roche cobas® EGFR mutation test v2 for non-small cell lung cancer. Expert Rev Mol Diagn 2017. https://doi.org/10.1080/14737159.2017.1288568.
25. Mok T, Wu YL, Lee JS, et al. Detection and dynamic changes of EGFR mutations from circulating tumor DNA as a predictor of survival outcomes in NSCLC Patients treated with first-line intercalated erlotinib and chemotherapy. Clin Cancer Res 2015.
26. Vogelstein B, Kinzler KW. Digital PCR. Genetics 1999;96:9236–41.
27. Garcia-Murillas I, Schiavon G, Weigelt B, et al. Mutation tracking in circulating tumor DNA predicts relapse in early breast cancer. Sci Transl Med 2015;7(302):1–7.
28. Oxnard GR, Thress KS, Alden RS, et al. Association between plasma genotyping and outcomes of treatment with osimertinib (AZD9291) in advanced non-small-cell lung cancer. J Clin Oncol 2016;34(28): 3375–82.
29. Sacher AG, Paweletz C, Dahlberg SE, et al. Prospective validation of rapid plasma genotyping as a sensitive and specific tool for guiding lung cancer care. JAMA Oncol 2016;2(8):1014–22.
30. Kinde I, Papadopoulos N, Kinzler KW, et al. FAST-SeqS: a simple and efficient method for the detection of aneuploidy by massively parallel sequencing. PLoS One 2012;7:1–8.
31. Leighl NB, Page RD, Raymond VM, et al. Clinical utility of comprehensive cell-free DNA analysis to identify genomic biomarkers in patients with newly diagnosed metastatic non-small cell lung cancer. Clin Cancer Res 2019. https://doi.org/10.1158/1078-0432.CCR-19-0624.
32. Abbosh C, Birkbak NJ, Swanton C. Early stage NSCLC: challenges to implementing ctDNA-based screening and MRD detection. Nat Rev Clin Oncol 2018. https://doi.org/10.1038/s41571-018-0058-3.
33. Newman AM, Lovejoy AF, Klass DM, et al. Integrated digital error suppression for improved detection of circulating tumor DNA. Nat Biotechnol 2016;34(5): 547–55.
34. Shagin DA, Shagina IA, Zaretsky AR, et al. A high-throughput assay for quantitative measurement of PCR errors. Sci Rep 2017;7(1):1–11.
35. Lindeman NI, Cagle PT, Aisner DL, et al. Updated molecular testing guideline for the selection of lung cancer patients for treatment with targeted tyrosine kinase inhibitors: guideline from the College of American Pathologists, the International Association for the Study of Lung Cancer, and the Association for Molecular Pathology. Arch Pathol Lab Med 2018. https://doi.org/10.5858/arpa.2017-0388-CP.
36. Zill OA, Banks KC, Fairclough SR, et al. The landscape of actionable genomic alterations in cell-free circulating tumor DNA from 21,807 advanced

cancer patients. Clin Cancer Res 2018;24(15): 3528–38.
37. Abbosh C, Birkbak NJ, Wilson GA, et al. Phylogenetic ctDNA analysis depicts early-stage lung cancer evolution. Nature 2017;545(7655):446–51.
38. Thress KS, Brant R, Carr TH, et al. EGFR mutation detection in ctDNA from NSCLC patient plasma: a cross-platform comparison of leading technologies to support the clinical development of AZD9291. Lung Cancer 2015;90(3):509–15.
39. Soria JC, Ohe Y, Vansteenkiste J, et al. Osimertinib in untreated EGFR-Mutated advanced non-small-cell lung cancer. N Engl J Med 2018. https://doi.org/10.1056/NEJMoa1713137.
40. Siravegna G, Marsoni S, Siena S, et al. Integrating liquid biopsies into the management of cancer. Nat Rev Clin Oncol 2017. https://doi.org/10.1038/nrclinonc.2017.14.
41. Hasan MM, Patel J, Johnson I, et al. Tracking minimal residual disease in post-operative cell-free DNA using MSK-ACCESS [abstract]. In: Proceedings of the American Association for Cancer Research Annual Meeting 2019; 2019 Mar 29-Apr 3; Atlanta, GA. Philadelphia (PA): AACR; Cancer Res 2019;79(13 Suppl):Abstract nr 1387.
42. Gale D, Lawson ARJ, Howarth K, et al. Development of a highly sensitive liquid biopsy platform to detect clinically-relevant cancer mutations at low allele fractions in cellfree DNA. PLoS One 2018. https://doi.org/10.1371/journal.pone.0194630.
43. Chabon JJ, Simmons AD, Lovejoy AF, et al. Analytical and clinical validation of a digital sequencing panel for quantitative, highly accurate evaluation of cell-free circulating tumor DNA. Clin Cancer Res 2017;545(5):60–5.
44. Sabari JK, Offin M, Stephens D, et al. A prospective study of circulating tumor DNA to guide matched targeted therapy in lung cancers. J Natl Cancer Inst 2019;111(6):575–83.
45. Gutierrez ME, Choi K, Lanman RB, et al. Genomic profiling of advanced non–small cell lung cancer in community settings: gaps and opportunities. Clin Lung Cancer 2017. https://doi.org/10.1016/j.cllc.2017.04.004.
46. Ettinger DS, Wood DE, Aisner DL, et al. Non–small cell lung cancer, version 5.2017, NCCN clinical practice guidelines in oncology. J Natl Compr Canc Netw 2017;15(4):504–35.
47. Chong CR, Jänne PA. The quest to overcome resistance to EGFR-targeted therapies in cancer. Nat Med 2013. https://doi.org/10.1038/nm.3388.
48. Jenkins S, Yang JCH, Ramalingam SS, et al. Plasma ctDNA analysis for detection of the EGFR T790M mutation in patients with advanced non–small cell lung cancer. J Thorac Oncol 2017. https://doi.org/10.1016/j.jtho.2017.04.003.
49. Gandara DR, Paul SM, Kowanetz M, et al. Blood-based tumor mutational burden as a predictor of clinical benefit in non-small-cell lung cancer patients treated with atezolizumab. Nat Med 2018. https://doi.org/10.1038/s41591-018-0134-3.
50. Fehrenbacher L, Spira A, Ballinger M, et al. Atezolizumab versus docetaxel for patients with previously treated non-small-cell lung cancer (POPLAR): a multicentre, open-label, phase 2 randomised controlled trial. Lancet 2016. https://doi.org/10.1016/S0140-6736(16)00587-0.
51. Rittmeyer A, Barlesi F, Waterkamp D, et al. Atezolizumab versus docetaxel in patients with previously treated non-small-cell lung cancer (OAK): a phase 3, open-label, multicentre randomised controlled trial. Lancet 2017;389(10066):255–65.
52. Goldberg SB, Narayan A, Kole AJ, et al. Early assessment of lung cancer immunotherapy response via circulating tumor DNA. Clin Cancer Res 2018;24(8):1872–80.
53. Nishino M, Jagannathan JP, Ramaiya NH, et al. Revised RECIST guideline version 1.1: what oncologists want to know and what radiologists need to know. Am J Roentgenol 2010;195(2): 281–9.
54. Kim EY, Cho EN, Park HS, et al. Genetic heterogeneity of actionable genes between primary and metastatic tumor in lung adenocarcinoma. BMC Cancer 2016. https://doi.org/10.1186/s12885-016-2049-z.
55. Jamal-Hanjani M, Hackshaw A, Ngai Y, et al. Tracking genomic cancer evolution for precision medicine: the lung TRACERx study. PLoS Biol 2014;12(7):1–7.
56. Jamal-Hanjani M, Wilson GA, McGranahan N, et al. Tracking the evolution of non–small-cell lung cancer. N Engl J Med 2017;376(22):2109–21.
57. Thress KS, Paweletz CP, Felip E, et al. Acquired EGFR C797S mutation mediates resistance to AZD9291 in non-small cell lung cancer harboring EGFR T790M. Nat Med 2015;21(6):560–2.
58. Phallen J, Sausen M, Adleff V, et al. Direct detection of early-stage cancers using circulating tumor DNA. Sci Transl Med 2017;9(403):1–12.
59. Chabon JJ, Simmons AD, Lovejoy AF, et al. Circulating tumour DNA profiling reveals heterogeneity of EGFR inhibitor resistance mechanisms in lung cancer patients. Nat Commun 2016;7: 1–14.
60. Tie J, Wang Y, Tomasetti C, et al. Circulating tumor DNA analysis detects minimal residual disease and predicts recurrence in patients with stage II colon cancer. Sci Transl Med 2016; 8(346):1–10.
61. Swanton C, Venn O, Aravanis A, et al. Prevalence of clonal hematopoiesis of indeterminate potential (CHIP) measured by an ultra-sensitive sequencing assay: exploratory analysis of the circulating cancer

genome atlas (CCGA) study. J Clin Oncol 2018; 36(15_suppl):12003.
62. Genovese G, Kähler AK, Handsaker RE, et al. Clonal hematopoiesis and blood-cancer risk inferred from blood DNA sequence. N Engl J Med 2014;371(26): 2477–87.
63. Jaiswal S, Fontanillas P, Flannick J, et al. Age-related clonal hematopoiesis associated with adverse outcomes. N Engl J Med 2014;371(26):2488–98.
64. Steensma DP, Bejar R, Jaiswal S, et al. Perspective: clonal hematopoiesis of indeterminate potential and its distinction from myelodysplastic syndromes. Blood 2018;126(4):9–17.
65. Acuna-Hidalgo R, Sengul H, Steehouwer M, et al. Ultra-sensitive sequencing identifies high prevalence of clonal hematopoiesis-associated mutations throughout adult life. Am J Hum Genet 2017; 101(1):50–64.
66. Zink F, Stacey SN, Norddahl GL, et al. Clonal hematopoiesis, with and without candidate driver mutations, is common in the elderly. Blood 2017;130(6): 742–52.
67. Young AL, Challen GA, Birmann BM, et al. Clonal haematopoiesis harbouring AML-associated mutations is ubiquitous in healthy adults. Nat Commun 2016;7:12484.
68. Bronkhorst AJ, Aucamp J, Pretorius PJ. Cell-free DNA: preanalytical variables. Clin Chim Acta 2015.
69. Underhill HR, Kitzman JO, Hellwig S, et al. Fragment length of circulating tumor DNA. PLoS Genet 2016; 12(7):1–24.
70. Mouliere F, Robert B, Peyrotte E, et al. High fragmentation characterizes tumour-derived circulating DNA. PLoS One 2011;6(9):e23418.
71. Mouliere F, Chandrananda D, Piskorz AM, et al. Enhanced detection of circulating tumor DNA by fragment size analysis. Sci Transl Med 2018; 10(466):1–14.
72. Xu T, Kang X, You X, et al. Cross-platform comparison of four leading technologies for detecting EGFR mutations in circulating tumor DNA from non-small cell lung carcinoma patient plasma. Theranostics 2017;7(6):1437–46.
73. Ye M, Li S, Huang W, et al. Comprehensive targeted super-deep next generation sequencing enhances differential diagnosis of solitary pulmonary nodules. J Thorac Dis 2018. https://doi.org/10.21037/jtd.2018.04.09.
74. Gettinger S, Horn L, Jackman D, et al. Five-year follow-up of nivolumab in previously treated advanced non–small-cell lung cancer: results from the CA209-003 study. J Clin Oncol 2018. https://doi.org/10.1200/JCO.2017.77.0412.
75. Krebs M, Dive C, Dean EJ, et al. TARGET trial: molecular profiling of circulating tumour DNA to stratify patients to early phase clinical trials. In: JCO ASCO meeting. Chicago, June 3–7, 2016. https://doi.org/10.1200/JCO.2016.34.15_suppl.TPS11614.

Adjuvant Chemotherapy

Jessica A. Hellyer, MD, Heather A. Wakelee, MD*

KEYWORDS

- Adjuvant • Chemotherapy • Targeted agents

KEY POINTS

- Standard of care for resectable, early-stage lung cancer is 4 cycles of adjuvant chemotherapy.
- Chemotherapy regimens have equitable efficacy, although in practice platinum plus pemetrexed is used most often for nonsquamous non–small cell lung cancer (NSCLC) due to favorable toxicity profile, with recent support for this approach from the JIPANG trial.
- Adjuvant immunotherapy is under investigation and discussed separately.
- Targeted therapies currently are not standard-of-care adjuvant treatment in driver mutation–positive early-stage NSCLC, but several trials are under way examining their use.

CHEMOTHERAPY

Introduction

More than 50% of patients with early-stage (I–III) non–small cell lung cancer (NSCLC) relapse within 5 years of surgical resection.[1] For patients with resectable stages II–IIIA disease at time of diagnosis, standard of care after surgery is 4 cycles of platinum-doublet chemotherapy.[2] Chemotherapy also may be considered in those patients with stage IB disease with high-risk features, such as poorly differentiated tumors, size greater than 4 cm, unknown lymph nodes status, vascular invasion, wedge resection, and visceral pleural involvement.[2] The overall benefit from chemotherapy, however, remains modest. In 2008, the Lung Adjuvant Cisplatin Evaluation group performed a pooled analysis of individual patient data from the largest cisplatin-based adjuvant trials performed since 1995, including 5 trials, with a total of 4584 patients. The primary endpoint was overall survival. There was a statistically significant reduction in mortality of 5.4% at 5 years in patients who received chemotherapy compared with those who did not (hazard ratio [HR] = 0.89; 95% CI, 0.82–0.96; P = .005).[1] This benefit was seen across all stages (IB, IIA, and IIB) with the exception of IA, although increased benefit was seen in those with higher stages of disease. In addition, the benefit from chemotherapy was the greatest in patients with Eastern Cooperative Oncology Group (ECOG) performance status (PS) of 0 and seemed to be detrimental to those patients with PS of 2. PS was not available, however, for all trials included in the analysis.[1] A follow-up meta-analysis in 2010 confirmed the benefits of adjuvant chemotherapy after evaluating 34 trials and 8447 patients and showing an increase in overall survival by 4% at 5 years with the addition of adjuvant chemotherapy.[3] Therefore, all patients with resected stages IB–IIIA disease should be referred to a medical oncologist for discussion of adjuvant chemotherapy.

Adjuvant Versus Neoadjuvant Chemotherapy

A meta-analysis published in 2009 compared the impact of timing of chemotherapy in patients with resectable lung cancer. They looked at 32 randomized trials, including 22 trials of adjuvant therapy and 10 trials of neoadjuvant therapy, and compared pooled HRs for death. The HR for overall survival was 0.80 (0.74–0.87; P<.001) in postoperative chemotherapy and 0.81 (0.68–0.97; P = .024) in preoperative chemotherapy. The secondary outcome, disease-free survival (DFS), was

Department of Medicine, Division of Oncology, Stanford Cancer Institute, Stanford University School of Medicine, 875 Blake Wilbur Drive, Stanford, CA 94305, USA
* Corresponding author.
E-mail address: hwakelee@stanford.edu

Thorac Surg Clin 30 (2020) 179–185
https://doi.org/10.1016/j.thorsurg.2020.01.003

compared between 15 postoperative and 7 preoperative chemotherapy trials and similarly did not show a difference between the 2 groups. The pooled HR for recurrence or death was 0.76 (0.68–0.85; *P*<.001) in postoperative chemotherapy and 0.80 (0.66–0.92; *P* = .021) in preoperative chemotherapy. Overall, the results demonstrate that there is no difference in DFS or overall survival between patients with operable lung cancer who receive postoperative versus preoperative chemotherapy.[4] At this time, with current chemotherapy options, adjuvant chemotherapy is preferable to neoadjuvant for patients who are surgically resectable at time of diagnosis in order to prevent delays in potentially curative surgical therapy.

Postoperative Complications

Many of the adjuvant chemotherapy trials excluded patients with severe postoperative complications and mandated chemotherapy initiation within 6 weeks to 9 weeks after surgery.[5,6] For patients with surgical complications who have a prolonged recovery period, however, the question of whether to give adjuvant chemotherapy outside the accepted window arises. Although this has not been evaluated in a randomized setting, real-world data from a retrospective analysis of 12,473 patients from the National Cancer Database suggest that these patients still benefit from chemotherapy. The study included patients with tumors greater than 4 cm, lymph node involvement, or local extension. The lowest mortality was observed in patients in whom chemotherapy was started within 50 days of resection. Approximately 30% of patients, however, received chemotherapy outside the accepted window (57–127 days postoperative) yet still had a survival benefit over patients who received surgery alone. Therefore, patients with a complicated postoperative course and prolonged recovery still may benefit from adjuvant chemotherapy up to 4 months after surgery.[7]

Choice of Chemotherapy

Acceptable choices for chemotherapy include a platinum backbone (generally cisplatin) with vinorelbine, pemetrexed, gemcitabine, or docetaxel.[8] In patients with metastatic NSCLC, comparison of cisplatin/paclitaxel, cisplatin/gemcitabine, cisplatin/docetaxel, and carboplatin/paclitaxel in a randomized study of 1207 patients with advanced NSCLC (stages IIIB–IV) failed to show a difference in survival between the 4 arms.[9] In the adjuvant setting, ECOG E1505 study also did not show a difference in outcome between chemotherapy doublets, although patients were not randomized to chemotherapy arm and the chemotherapy doublet utilized was not the primary question. In this study, 1500 patients were randomized to chemotherapy plus bevacizumab versus chemotherapy alone. The chemotherapy regimen was investigator's choice and included cisplatin paired with gemcitabine, pemetrexed, vinorelbine, or docetaxel. Although the study was not powered to compare the chemotherapy regimens, a subset analysis showed similar efficacy between platinum doublets in the chemotherapy arm.[10]

Pemetrexed, a folate analog, was developed later than the taxanes gemcitabine and vinorelbine but quickly was adopted into practice for nonsquamous NSCLC given its favorable toxicity profile.[11] In the metastatic setting, a randomized phase III study of cisplatin/gemcitabine versus cisplatin/pemetrexed showed that overall survival was superior for pemetrexed in the nonsquamous arm (12.6 months vs 10.9 months) and that it is better tolerated than gemcitabine. Pemetrexed is not approved for patients with squamous histology, however, because overall survival was inferior to cisplatin/gemcitabine.[12] Given the tolerability profile and early data from the phase II TREAT study, cisplatin/pemetrexed has been widely adopted in the adjuvant setting and was in fact the regimen used in the largest number of patients on E1505 despite that it was limited to patients with nonsquamous histology and was added to the trial only after enrollment had been ongoing for 2 years. More recently, the Japan Intergroup Trial of Pemetrexed Adjuvant Chemotherapy for Completely Resected Nonsquamous Non-Small-Cell Lung Cancer (JIPANG) study gave us clear randomized phase III data to support the use of cisplatin/pemetrexed in the adjuvant setting. JIPANG was a phase III study of cisplatin/pemetrexed compared with cisplatin/vinorelbine for resected, stages II–IIIA, nonsquamous lung cancer. The study enrolled 804 patients and at a follow-up of 45 months there was no significant difference between the 2 treatment arms with a median recurrence free survival of 38.9 months in the cisplatin/pemetrexed cohort and 37.3 months in the cisplatin/vinorelbine cohort (HR 0.98; 95% CI, 0.81–1.2; *P* = .948).[6] Overall survival was also similar between the 2 arms (83.5% cisplatin/pemetrexed vs 87.2% cisplatin/vinorelbine). Similar to prior studies, however, they also found that cisplatin/pemetrexed was less toxic and better tolerated than cisplatin/vinorelbine.[6]

Although cisplatin is the preferred platinum agent in the adjuvant setting, its toxicity profile precludes use in many patients. Nephrotoxicity and ototoxicity top the list of adverse events, and it must be used cautiously in elderly patients and those with significant comorbidities. Due to these toxicities, carboplatin, which is mechanistically similar to cisplatin but generally better tolerated, often is substituted for cisplatin in frail or elderly patients. A Cochrane review examined the evidence from randomized clinical trials comparing carboplatin with cisplatin plus a partner drug in patients with advanced NSCLC. They included 10 trials with 5017 patients and found that there was no difference in overall survival between those patients who received carboplatin and those who received cisplatin (HR 1.0; 95% CI, 0.51–1.97).[13] Few prospective trials, however, utilized carboplatin and caution must be taken in using carboplatin given a potential detriment in efficacy. Thus, although carboplatin is a reasonable substitution for patients unable to tolerate cisplatin-based chemotherapy, it should not be used routinely in those who can tolerate cisplatin.

Chemotherapy Combinations

Attempts to improve outcomes in early-stage patients treated with adjuvant chemotherapy led to trials adding targeted agents to chemotherapy. The E1505 examined the impact of bevacizumab, an anti–vascular endothelial growth factor (VEGF) agent on overall survival in patients with resected stages IB (>4 cm) to IIIA NSCLC. Patients were randomized to 4 cycles of chemotherapy alone (investigators choice—cisplatin plus vinorelbine, docetaxel, gemcitabine, or pemetrexed) or chemotherapy plus 1 year of bevacizumab. At a follow-up of 50 months, there was no difference in DFS (HR 0.98; P = .75) or overall survival (HR 0.99; P = .90).[10] Therefore, bevacizumab is not given in the adjuvant setting.

Patient Selection

Improving patient selection remains an important goal of ongoing chemotherapy trials, because not all patients need adjuvant chemotherapy, yet the ability to select for those who will benefit remains difficult. ERCC1, a protein involved in DNA repair pathways, was examined retrospectively in a cohort of patients enrolled in the International Adjuvant Lung Cancer Trial. They found that expression of this protein was associated with shorter survival and lack of benefit to adjuvant chemotherapy compared with ERCC1-negative tumors.[14] This was followed by a randomized phase II trial that enrolled 150 patients with resected NSCLC tumors and randomized patients to standard-of-care chemotherapy versus customized treatment based on ERCC1 levels (ie those ERCC1-negative patients received chemotherapy and positive patients went on observation). This trial had to be stopped, however, due to the unreliability of the ERCC1 stain, which also invalidated the earlier observations and stopped use of ERCC1 as a reliable biomarker.[15] Other potential biomarkers for chemotherapy selection include BRCA1, RAP80,[16] and ABRX.[17] In the Study of Customized Adjuvant Chemotherapy (SCAT) trial, patients were assigned to 1 of 3 adjuvant chemotherapy arms based on expression of BRCA1; patients with low expression received cisplatin/gemcitabine, with intermediate expression received cisplatin/docetaxel, and with high expression received docetaxel alone. At a follow-up of 5 years, there were similar DFS and overall survival rates between the cohorts.[18] To date, no biomarkers have been validated for patient selection of adjuvant chemotherapy.

Circulating tumor DNA (ctDNA) identification of minimal residual disease (MRD) has emerged as a potential tool to improve patient selection. A retrospective study of 40 patients with localized lung cancer found that those patients with detectable ctDNA MRD after curative therapy were highly likely to recur (freedom from progression at 36 months: 93% in patients with undetectable ctDNA MRD and 0% in patients with detectable ctDNA).[19] ctDNA is still under investigation, and there are several ongoing trials using MRD to either select patients for adjuvant chemotherapy or provide escalated treatment to those patients with MRD after completion of standard adjuvant therapy.[20]

IMMUNOTHERAPY

There are several adjuvant and neoadjuvant immunotherapy studies under way with promising results reported from the ongoing neoadjuvant studies at the American Society of Clinical Oncology 2019 annual meeting, with data on the adjuvant studies pending. The role of immunotherapy in this patient population and preliminary data are discussed later.

TARGETED THERAPY

Vaccine Trials

The MAGRIT (MAGE-A3 as Adjuvant Non-Small Cell Lung Cancer Immunotherapy) trial was a randomized, double-blind, placebo-controlled, phase II study of MAGE-A3 (melanoma associated antigen 3) vaccine in patients with resected stages IB, II or IIIA NSCLC whose tumors expressed MAGE-A3; 2312 patients were enrolled in the study and randomized 2:1 to 13 injections of the MAGE-A3 vaccine versus placebo. Patients were allowed to have received adjuvant chemotherapy but it was not mandated. There were 3 coprimary endpoints: DFS in all-comers, DFS in the no-chemotherapy group, and DFS in patients stratified by potentially predictive gene signature. In all patients, the DFS was 60.5 months in the MAGE-A3 arm and 57.9 in the placebo group (HR 1.02; 95% CI, 0.89–1.18; *P* = .74). Similarly, in the no-chemotherapy arm, DFS was 58 months in the MAGE-A3 group compared with 56.9 in the placebo group (HR 0.97; 95% CI, 0.80–1.18; *P* = .76).[21] Given the negative study, no other trials have been conducted with this compound. Other therapeutic vaccine trials in NSCLC have largely been conducted in patients with unresectable stages IIIB–IV disease.[22]

Epidermal Growth Factor Receptor–Tyrosine Kinase Inhibitor in Unselected Patients

Early studies looking at adjuvant epidermal growth factor receptor (EGFR)–tyrosine kinase inhibitors (TKIs) were performed in an unselected patient population. Gefinitib was examined in the cooperative group BR19 study in stage IB, II, or IIIA patients after surgical resection and adjuvant chemotherapy; 503 patients were enrolled and randomized to gefinitib versus placebo for 2 years. The study closed early, however, after a median of 4.7 years of follow-up after an interim analysis failed to show a difference in DFS or overall survival. Exploratory analysis of the patients with EGFR mutation–positive tumors (N = 15 [4%]) also did not show a benefit in DFS (HR 1.84; 95% CI, 0.44–7.73; *P* = .395) or overall survival (HR 3.16; 95% CI, 0.61–16.45; *P* = .15) although this was a small subset (15 patients) of the overall cohort.[23]

Epidermal Growth Factor Receptor–Tyrosine Kinase Inhibitors in Selected Patients

After trials of EGFR-TKIs in unselected patients failed to show a benefit, additional studies selecting patients for EGFR mutation or overexpression were developed as the understanding of EGFR biology improved. The RADIANT trial was a randomized, double-blind phase III trial of erlotinib versus placebo for 2 years after resection of stages IB–IIIA NSCLC. Patients were included if their tumor expressed EGFR protein by immunohistochemistry or amplification by fluorescence in situ hybridization. A total of 973 patients were enrolled. Similar to the trials in an unselected cohort of patients, this trial failed to show a difference in DFS (median 50.5 months for erlotinib and 48.2 months for placebo; *P* = .324) or overall survival (HR 1.13; 95% CI, 0.881–1.448; *P* = .3350). There was a subgroup of patients, however, with L858R and exon 19 deletion EGFR-mutant tumors (n = 161); 102 were assigned to erlotinib and 59 to placebo. In this subgroup, there was a trend toward improvement in DFS but due to hierarchical testing this difference was not statistically significant (DFS 28.5 months in placebo vs 48.2 months in erlotinib arm; HR 0.61; 95% CI, 0.384–0.981).[24]

A nonrandomized phase II trial of adjuvant erlotinib (SELECT trial) in patients with resected stages IA to IIIA EGFR-mutant NSCLC also was conducted and reported. A total of 100 patients were enrolled and treated with erlotinib daily for 2 years after standard adjuvant chemotherapy. The data are still immature but the 5-year DFS was recently reported out at 56% (95% CI, 45%–66%) and 5-year overall survival was 86% (95% CI, 77%–92%).[25]

The largest phase III trial of adjuvant EGFR-TKI to date in a selected patient population was the ADJUVANT/CTONG1104 study. As opposed to the other trials that randomized or treated patients with EGFR-TKI after completion of adjuvant chemotherapy, this multi-institutional, randomized, phase III study in China randomized patients to adjuvant gefitinib or chemotherapy. In this study, 222 patients with exon 19 deletion or exon 21 L858R EGFR mutated stages II–IIIA lung adenocarcinoma were enrolled and randomized 1:1 to gefitinib for 2 years or 4 cycles of vinorelbine/cisplatin after surgical resection. Median DFS was 28.7 months in the gefitinib arm compared with 18 months in the chemotherapy arm (HR 0.60; 95% CI, 0.42–0.87; *P* = .0054). Survival data are not yet available and, therefore, it is not clear whether adjuvant gefitinib given for 2 years simply delays disease recurrence without improving the overall cure rate.[26]

Epidermal Growth Factor Receptor–Tyrosine Kinase Inhibitor in the Neoadjuvant and Adjuvant Setting

A multicenter, randomized, open-label, phase II study of erlotinib versus chemotherapy as both neoadjuvant and adjuvant treatment in China was recently reported; 72 patients with EGFR mutations in either exon 19 or exon 21 were randomized 1:1 to receive erlotinib for 42 days prior to surgery and up to 12 months postoperatively or cisplatin/gemcitabine for 2 cycles prior to surgery and 2 cycles postoperatively. The primary endpoint was objective response rate. The study did not meet its primary endpoint (overall response rate 54.1 vs 34.3%; odds ratio 2.26; 95% CI, 0.87–5.84; *P* = .092). The secondary endpoint of progression-free survival was noted to be better for the erlotinib arm compared with the chemotherapy arm (21.5 months vs 11.4 months; HR 0.39; 95% CI, 0.23–0.67; *P*<.001); however, there was no difference in overall survival (45.8 vs 39.2 months; HR 0.77; 95% CI, 0.41–1.45; $P = .417$).[27] Although this study was small and did not meet its primary endpoint, there are several, larger ongoing randomized trials examining EGFR therapies in the adjuvant setting (discussed later).

Ongoing Targeted Adjuvant Studies

With the promising data from the targeted adjuvant studies in NSCLC, several large randomized trials have opened in selected patient populations. Icotinib, an EGFR-targeted agent, is being examined in several adjuvant studies. The EVIDENCE trial (NCT02448797) is a randomized, phase III study in China in patients with resected stages II–IIIA NSCLC with EGFR mutations. In this study, approximately 320 patients are randomized 1:1 to receive adjuvant icotinib for up to 2 years or 4 cycles of platinum-doublet chemotherapy. Crossover is allowed because patients in the chemotherapy arm will be provided free icotinib after completion of chemotherapy.[28] The ICTAN (NCT01996098) is a phase III study that randomizes patients with EGFR-mutant, stages II-IIIA NSCLC to icotinib versus observation following completion of adjuvant chemotherapy. Patients can be randomized to one of two icotinib arms to receive treatment for 6 or 12 months. Primary endpoint is DFS. Finally, the ICWIP study (NCT02125240) is a randomized phase III study of icotinib versus placebo for patients with EGFR-mutant, resected stages II–IIIA NSCLC. Primary outcome is DFS. As of the last update, all 3 studies currently are recruiting.

In Japan, the IMPACT WJOG6410L study is under way examining gefitinib versus chemotherapy as adjuvant therapy in patients with resected stages II–III NSCLC with activating EGFR mutations. Patients are randomized 1:1 to gefitinib for up to 2 years or 4 cycles of vinorelbine/cisplatin. The primary endpoint is DFS.[29]

The ALCHEMIST trial (NCT02194738) currently is recruiting patients with stages IB–IIIA NSCLC in the United States. Up to 8000 patients may be enrolled in the screening portion of the study. After surgical resection and standard-of-care adjuvant chemotherapy, patients are placed in 1 of 3 treatment arms based off of their tumor's driver mutation status. Patients with EGFR-mutant tumors are randomized to receive adjuvant erlotinib for up to 2 years versus placebo. Those with anaplastic lymphoma kinase (ALK)positive tumors are randomized to up to 2 years of crizotinib versus placebo. Finally, those patients without EGFR or ALK mutations will be randomized to up to 1 year of adjuvant nivolumab versus placebo. Coprimary endpoints are DFS and overall survival.[30]

The ADAURA study (NCT02511106) is a multicenter, double-blind, randomized, placebo-controlled trial of osimertinib, a third-generation EGFR-TKI, versus placebo. This study has finished recruiting with results anticipated in the next couple years. Patients with stages IB–IIIA NSCLC with exon 19 deletion or L858R mutation were enrolled after surgical resection; patients were allowed to receive postoperative chemotherapy but it was not mandated. They were randomized 1:1 to up to 3 years of osimertinib versus placebo. Primary endpoint is DFS; although, with any adjuvant trial, the overall survival is truly the critical outcome that would be practice-changing.[31] The data from RADIANT have shown that a DFS benefit may not translate into overall survival benefit if the EGFR-TKI therapy is only postponing but not preventing development of metastatic disease in this setting.

SUMMARY

At this time, standard of care for patients with resected stages IB (>4 cm)–IIIA disease remains 4 cycles of adjuvant platinum-doublet chemotherapy. Patients benefit modestly, however, from chemotherapy with an average improvement in overall survival of 5% at 5 years. Attempts to improve this by developing new chemotherapy combinations or adding anti-VEGF agents to chemotherapy were not successful. The trials of EGFR-targeted therapies held promise but also did not show a benefit in an unselected patient population. Studies of EGFR-targeted therapies in patients with EGFR driver mutations, however, showed a possible signal of efficacy. As a result, rigorous studies examining EGFR and ALK-targeted agents in patients with driver mutation NSCLC currently are ongoing and results are eagerly awaited.

DISCLOSURE

Dr H.A. Wakelee: honoraria from Novartis and AstraZeneca; advisory board participation (compensated): AstraZeneca and Xcovery; advisory board (NOT compensated): Merck, Takeda, and Genentech/Roche; research funding to institution: ACEA Biosciences, Arrys Therapeutics, AstraZeneca/Medimmune, Bayer, BMS, Celgene, Clovis Oncology, Exelixis, Genentech/Roche, Gilead, Lilly, Merck, Novartis, Pfizer, Pharmacyclics, and Xcovery; and travel: AstraZeneca. Dr J.A. Hellyer has no relevant conflicts of interest to disclose.

REFERENCES

1. Pignon JP, Tribodet H, Scagliotti GV, et al. Lung adjuvant cisplatin evaluation: a pooled analysis by the LACE collaborative group. J Clin Oncol 2008; 26(21):3552–9.
2. National Comprehensive Cancer Network. Non-small cell lung cancer version 4. 2019. Available at: https://www.nccn.org/professionals/physician_gls/pdf/nscl.pdf. Accessed August 22, 2019.
3. Arriagada R, Auperin A, Burdett S, et al. Adjuvant chemotherapy, with or without postoperative radiotherapy, in operable non-small-cell lung cancer: two meta-analyses of individual patient data. Lancet 2010;375(9722):1267–77.
4. Lim E, Harris G, Patel A, et al. Preoperative versus postoperative chemotherapy in patients with resectable non-small cell lung cancer: systematic review and indirect comparison meta-analysis of randomized trials. J Thorac Oncol 2009;4(11): 1380–8.
5. Douillard JY, Rosell R, De Lena M, et al. Adjuvant vinorelbine plus cisplatin versus observation in patients with completely resected stage IB-IIIA non-small-cell lung cancer (Adjuvant Navelbine International Trialist Association [ANITA]): a randomised controlled trial. Lancet Oncol 2006;7(9):719–27.
6. Yamamoto N, Kenmotsu H, Yamanaka T, et al. Randomized phase III study of cisplatin with pemetrexed and cisplatin with vinorelbine for completely resected nonsquamous non-small-cell lung cancer: the JIPANG study protocol. Clin Lung Cancer 2018;19(1):e1–3.
7. Salazar MC, Rosen JE, Wang Z, et al. Association of delayed adjuvant chemotherapy with survival after lung cancer surgery. JAMA Oncol 2017;3(5):610–9.
8. National Comprehensive Cancer Network. NCCN guidelines version 5.2019. Non-small cell lung cancer 2019.
9. Schiller JH, Harrington D, Belani CP, et al. Comparison of four chemotherapy regimens for advanced non-small-cell lung cancer. N Engl J Med 2002; 346(2):92–8.
10. Wakelee HA, Dahlberg SE, Keller SM, et al. Adjuvant chemotherapy with or without bevacizumab in patients with resected non-small-cell lung cancer (E1505): an open-label, multicentre, randomised, phase 3 trial. Lancet Oncol 2017;18(12): 1610–23.
11. Kreuter M, Vansteenkiste J, Fischer JR, et al. Randomized phase 2 trial on refinement of early-stage NSCLC adjuvant chemotherapy with cisplatin and pemetrexed versus cisplatin and vinorelbine: the TREAT study. Ann Oncol 2013;24(4):986–92.
12. Scagliotti GV, Parikh P, von Pawel J, et al. Phase III study comparing cisplatin plus gemcitabine with cisplatin plus pemetrexed in chemotherapy-naive patients with advanced-stage non-small-cell lung cancer. J Clin Oncol 2008;26(21):3543–51.
13. de Castria TB, da Silva EM, Gois AF, et al. Cisplatin versus carboplatin in combination with third-generation drugs for advanced non-small cell lung cancer. Cochrane Database Syst Rev 2013;(8): CD009256.
14. Olaussen KA, Dunant A, Fouret P, et al. DNA repair by ERCC1 in non-small-cell lung cancer and cisplatin-based adjuvant chemotherapy. N Engl J Med 2006;355(10):983–91.
15. Wislez M, Barlesi F, Besse B, et al. Customized adjuvant phase II trial in patients with non-small-cell lung cancer: IFCT-0801 TASTE. J Clin Oncol 2014;32(12): 1256–61.
16. Rosell R, Perez-Roca L, Sanchez JJ, et al. Customized treatment in non-small-cell lung cancer based on EGFR mutations and BRCA1 mRNA expression. PLoS One 2009;4(5):e5133.
17. Joerger M, deJong D, Burylo A, et al. Tubulin, BRCA1, ERCC1, Abraxas, RAP80 mRNA expression, p53/p21 immunohistochemistry and clinical outcome in patients with advanced non small-cell lung cancer receiving first-line platinum-gemcitabine chemotherapy. Lung Cancer 2011;74(2): 310–7.
18. Massuti B, Cobo M, Rodriguez-Paniagua M. SCAT Ph III trial: adjuvant CT based on BRCA1 levels in NSCLC N+ resected patients. Final survival results a spanish lung cancer group trial. J Thorac Oncol 2017;(12):S1605.
19. Chaudhuri AA, Chabon JJ, Lovejoy AF, et al. Early detection of molecular residual disease in localized lung cancer by circulating tumor DNA profiling. Cancer Discov 2017;7(12):1394–403.
20. Coakley M, Garcia-Murillas I, Turner NC. Molecular residual disease and adjuvant trials design in solid tumors. Clin Cancer Res 2019;25(20):6026–34.
21. Vansteenkiste JF, Cho BC, Vanakesa T, et al. Efficacy of the MAGE-A3 cancer immunotherapeutic as adjuvant therapy in patients with resected MAGE-A3-positive non-small-cell lung cancer (MAGRIT): a randomised, double-blind, placebo-controlled, phase 3 trial. Lancet Oncol 2016;17(6): 822–35.
22. Socola F, Scherfenberg N, Raez LE. Therapeutic vaccines in non-small cell lung cancer. Immunotargets Ther 2013;2:115–24.
23. Goss GD, O'Callaghan C, Lorimer I, et al. Gefitinib versus placebo in completely resected non-small-cell lung cancer: results of the NCIC CTG BR19 study. J Clin Oncol 2013;31(27):3320–6.
24. Kelly K, Altorki NK, Eberhardt WE, et al. Adjuvant erlotinib versus placebo in patients with stage IB-IIIA non-small-cell lung cancer (RADIANT): a randomized, double-blind, phase III trial. J Clin Oncol 2015;33(34):4007–14.

25. Pennell NA, Neal JW, Chaft JE, et al. SELECT: a phase II trial of adjuvant erlotinib in patients with resected epidermal growth factor receptor-mutant non-small-cell lung cancer. J Clin Oncol 2019; 37(2):97–104.
26. Zhong WZ, Wang Q, Mao WM, et al. Gefitinib versus vinorelbine plus cisplatin as adjuvant treatment for stage II-IIIA (N1-N2) EGFR-mutant NSCLC (ADJUVANT/CTONG1104): a randomised, open-label, phase 3 study. Lancet Oncol 2018;19(1):139–48.
27. Zhong WZ, Chen KN, Chen C, et al. Erlotinib versus gemcitabine plus cisplatin as neoadjuvant treatment of stage IIIA-N2 EGFR-mutant non-small-cell lung cancer (EMERGING-CTONG 1103): a randomized phase II study. J Clin Oncol 2019;37(25): 2235–45.
28. He J, Liang W, Xu S, et al. Icotinib versus vinorelbine/platinum as adjuvant therapy in stage II-IIIA non-small cell lung cancer with EGFR-mutations: a multicenter, randomized, positive-controlled, phase 3, indication-expanding study (EVIDENCE, CCTC-1501). J Clin Oncol 2016;4:15(suppl, TPS8570-TPS8570).
29. Tada H, Takeda K, Nakagawa K, et al. Vinorelbine plus cisplatin versus gefitinib in resected non-small cell lung cancer haboring activating EGFR mutation (WJOG6410L). J Clin Oncol 2012;30:TPS7110.
30. Govindan R, Mandrekar SJ, Gerber DE, et al. ALCHEMIST trials: a golden opportunity to transform outcomes in early-stage non-small cell lung cancer. Clin Cancer Res 2015;21(24):5439–44.
31. Wu YL, Herbst RS, Mann H, et al. ADAURA: phase III, double-blind, randomized study of osimertinib versus placebo in EGFR mutation-positive early-stage NSCLC after complete surgical resection. Clin Lung Cancer 2018;19(4):e533–6.

Principles of Immunotherapy in Non-Small Cell Lung Cancer

Melinda L. Hsu, MD[a,*], Jarushka Naidoo, MBBCH, MHS[b]

KEYWORDS

• Immune checkpoint inhibitors • Immunotherapy • Non-small cell lung cancer • Anti-PD-1
• Anti-PD-L1

KEY POINTS

- Immune checkpoint inhibitors (ICI) remove the blockade of T cell activation caused by tumor cells, thereby unleashing the immune system.
- ICI are FDA approved for the treatment of both treatment-naive and previously treated patients with advanced NSCLC, and also as maintenance after chemoradiotherapy in stage IIII NSCLC.
- Key areas of ongoing research include identification of predictive biomarkers of response, such as the gut microbiome, and the use of ICIs in earlier disease settings.

INTRODUCTION

Immune checkpoint inhibitors (ICI) are a novel class of drugs which have the ability to restore antitumor T cell responses by blocking inhibition of T cell activation in the tumor microenvironment and beyond.[1,2] Ipilimumab was the first ICI to receive Food and Drug Administration (FDA) approval in 2011 for the treatment of metastatic melanoma,[3] and ICIs were subsequently evaluated for efficacy in the treatment of multiple other tumor types.[4] In particular, anti-PD-1/PD-L1 ICIs have transformed the landscape of therapy for patients with non-small cell lung cancer (NSCLC), and now form part of the standard treatment armamentarium in both stage III[5,6] and stage IV[7–9] NSCLC. In this review, we provide a brief summary of the mechanism of action of ICIs, the clinical data that support current use of ICIs in the treatment of NSCLC, and a brief discussion of future directions in the field.

How Do Immune Checkpoint Inhibitors Work?

ICIs allow for T cells to mount an antitumor response by overcoming the normal regulatory mechanisms of T cell activation. Tumor cells express tumor-specific antigens in the context of the major histocompatibility complex, which are presented on antigen-presenting cells (APCs), allowing the T cell to recognize the tumor. A second signal is needed to activate the T cell, which involves the CD28 receptor on T cells engaging with the B7 receptor (CD80/86) on the APC. T cell activation is actually more complex, however, as it also induces an inhibitory pathway that provides self-regulation by either attenuating or abrogating the T cell response. T cells express immune checkpoint molecules, such as cytotoxic T lymphocyte-associated antigen 4 (CTLA-4) and programmed cell death protein 1 (PD-1), which are upregulated on T cell activation. CTLA-4 downregulates T cell activation by outcompeting

[a] Department of Oncology, Sidney Kimmel Comprehensive Cancer Center, Bloomberg-Kimmel Institute for Cancer Immunotherapy, Johns Hopkins University, 1650 Orleans Street CRB1 186, Baltimore, MD 21287, USA; [b] Department of Oncology, Sidney Kimmel Comprehensive Cancer Center, Bloomberg-Kimmel Institute for Cancer Immunotherapy, Johns Hopkins University, 401 North Broadway, Baltimore, MD 21287, USA
* Corresponding author.
E-mail address: Mhsu14@jhmi.edu
Twitter: @DrJNaidoo (J.N.)

Thorac Surg Clin 30 (2020) 187–198
https://doi.org/10.1016/j.thorsurg.2020.01.009
1547-4127/20/

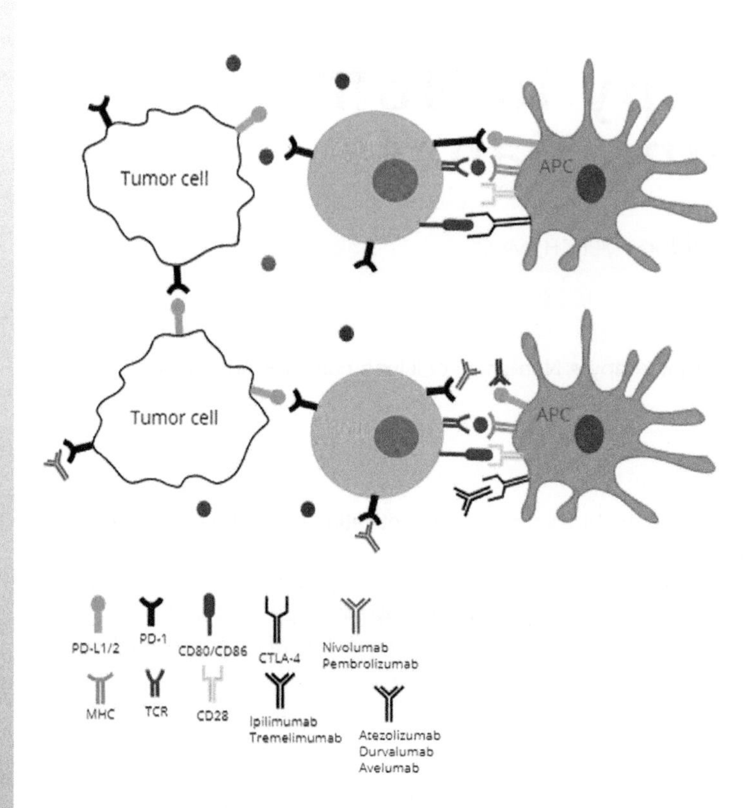

Fig. 1. Mechanism of action of immune checkpoint inhibitors.

CD28 for B7 (CD80/86) and inducing T cell cycle arrest, thus decreasing T cell activation.[10,11] The hypothesis that an antibody against CTLA-4 would block its interaction with B7 and consequently allow sufficient T cell responses to increase antitumor activity was demonstrated in mice[12] and led to the development of ipilimumab, which ultimately because the first FDA-approved ICI granted for the treatment of metastatic melanoma.[13]

After the clinical success of CTLA-4, other immune checkpoint molecules were targeted, including PD-1. PD-1 is expressed on several immunologic cells, including B cells, natural killer cells, and monocytes, and, unlike CTLA-4, directly regulates T cell activation.[14] Activation of T and B lymphocytes leads to expression of PD-1,[15] which binds to its ligands PD-L1 and PD-L2. PD-L1 and PD-L2 are expressed in response to inflammatory cytokines, and when PD-1 binds to them it inhibits the kinase signaling pathway that ordinarily activates T cells.[16] This helps protect against autoimmunity in the normal immune milieu, but also allows for tumors to evade the immune system, as PD-L1 and PD-L2 can both be expressed on tumor cells.[17] Blockade of PD-1 or its ligand PD-L1 removes this negative signal and, as the ligands are widely expressed in nonlymphoid tissues, restores the antitumor T cell response in the periphery (**Fig. 1**).[18]

CLINICAL DATA OF ANTI-PD-1/PD-L1 MONOTHERAPY IN NON-SMALL CELL LUNG CANCER

Nivolumab

Nivolumab, a fully human immunoglobulin G4 (IgG4) monoclonal antibody against PD-1, was the first ICI granted FDA approval for chemotherapy-treated NSCLC. It was approved in 2015 based on a randomized, open-label, international, phase III study (CheckMate-017) comparing nivolumab versus docetaxel[19] in previously treated patients with advanced squamous NSCLC (n = 272). At the pre-planned interim analysis, overall survival (OS), 1-year OS, and objective response rate (ORR) all statistically significantly favored nivolumab, leading to early closure of the trial. Median OS was 9.2 months in the nivolumab group (95% CI: 7.3–13.3) versus 6.0 months in the docetaxel group (95% CI: 5.1–7.3); hazard ratio (HR) was 0.59 (95% CI: 0.44–0.79; $P<.001$); and the 1-year OS with nivolumab of 42% was significantly higher than with docetaxel of 24%. In addition, progression-free survival (PFS) at 1 year was 21% (95% CI: 14–28) in nivolumab and 6% (95% CI: 3–12) in docetaxel. Treatment-related adverse events (AEs) were less frequent in the nivolumab group (58% of any grade) than the docetaxel group (86% of any grade), and led to treatment discontinuation less frequently in nivolumab (3% of patients) than in docetaxel (10% of patients), as per **Table 1**.

Nivolumab was concurrently evaluated in patients with previously treated, advanced, nonsquamous NSCLC (n = 582) in a randomized, open-label, international, phase III study (CheckMate-057),[20] again compared with standard second-line docetaxel. The pre-planned interim analysis revealed statistical significance in OS, 1-year OS, and ORR in favor of nivolumab, which led to early closure of the trial. Median OS was 13.2 months in the nivolumab group (95% CI: 9.7–10.5) and 9.4 months in the docetaxel group (95% CI: 8.1–10.7), with HR of 0.73 (95% CI: 0.59–0.89, *P* = .002). The 1-year OS for nivolumab was 51% compared with 39% for docetaxel. ORR for nivolumab of 19% was significantly higher than for docetaxel of 12%. Although median PFS for nivolumab was 2.3 months versus 4.2 months for docetaxel, the 1-year PFS for nivolumab was 19% versus 8% for docetaxel. There were fewer grade 3+ AEs in the nivolumab group (10%) than in the docetaxel group (54%). Discontinuation of treatment was less frequent with nivolumab (5%) than with docetaxel (15%). These results led to expansion of FDA approval for second-line monotherapy with nivolumab for advanced nonsquamous NSCLC (see **Table 1**).

Pembrolizumab

Pembrolizumab is a humanized IgG4 monoclonal antibody against PD-1, which was first evaluated in a phase 1 trial in advanced melanoma. In this study, pembrolizumab monotherapy demonstrated a 38% ORR and overall median PFS that was not greater than 7 months.[21] In NSCLC a subsequent international phase 1 trial (Keynote-001) evaluated pembrolizumab in both previously treated and previously untreated patients (n = 495) at 3 different dose levels: 2 mg/kg every 3 weeks, 10 mg/kg every 3 weeks, or 10 mg/kg every 2 weeks.[22] ORR was similar across dose, schedule, and tumor histology analyses, with an ORR of 19.4% (95% CI: 16.0–23.2). This included an 18.0% response rate in previously treated patients and 24.8% response rate in previously untreated patients. Median duration of response (DOR) was 12.5 months for all patients, with 84.4% of patients who had a response without disease progression. Median OS was 12.0 months for all patients. The trial also evaluated PD-L1 immunohistochemical (IHC) expression as a potential predictive biomarker of response, and in patients with PD-L1 expression of at least 50%, ORR was 45.2% (95% CI: 33.5–57.3). As a result, not only did pembrolizumab receive FDA approval as second-line monotherapy treatment of PD-L1-positive advanced NSCLC, but the companion diagnostic PD-L1 IHC 22C3 pharmDx test was also approved.

The success of Keynote-001 led to a subsequent phase II/III trial (Keynote-010), which evaluated pembrolizumab in patients with previously treated PD-L1-positive (tumor proportion score greater than 1%) NSCLC (n = 1034) at 2 doses, 2 or 10 mg/kg, versus docetaxel.[23] The primary endpoints of OS and PFS were evaluated, with a concurrent goal to validate the 22C3 biomarker with a PD-L1 cutoff score of ≥50%. In the total population, median OS was significantly improved for both doses of pembrolizumab at 10.4 months in the 2-mg/kg group (95% CI: 9.4–11.9), 12.7 months in the 10 mg/kg group (95% CI: 10.0–17.3), and 8.5 months versus docetaxel. In the patients with ≥50% PD-L1 expression, PFS was significantly longer with HR of 0.59 (*P* = .0001) for pembrolizumab 2 mg/kg versus docetaxel, and also HR of 0.59 (*P*<.0001) for pembrolizumab 10 mg/kg versus docetaxel. More impressively, median OS for the group of patients with greater than 50% PD-L1 expression was 14.9 months in the pembrolizumab 2 mg/kg group (95% CI: 10.4–not reached), 17.3 months in the pembrolizumab 10 mg/kg group (95% CI: 11.8–not reached), and 8.2 months in the docetaxel group (see **Table 1**). Grade 3+ treatment-related AEs were highest in the docetaxel group at 35% compared with 13% in the pembrolizumab 2 mg/kg group and 16% in the pembrolizumab 10 mg/kg group.

These data also supported the investigation of pembrolizumab monotherapy in a first-line phase III trial of patients with metastatic NSCLC (n = 305) with PD-L1 expression ≥50% (Keynote-024) comparing pembrolizumab (200 mg fixed dose) to platinum chemotherapy of the investigator's choice.[24] In this practice-changing study, the median PFS was 10.3 months (95% CI: 6.7–not reached) in the pembrolizumab group, and 6.0 months in the chemotherapy group, with HR of 0.50 (95% CI: 0.37–0.68, *P*<.001). OS was significantly prolonged with an HR of 0.60 (95% CI: 0.41–0.89, *P* = .005), and estimated OS at 6 months 80.2% with pembrolizumab versus 72.4% with chemotherapy. This led to early closure of the trial to allow patients in the chemotherapy arm to receive pembrolizumab, as well as FDA approval for pembrolizumab as first-line monotherapy in patients with PD-L1 expression ≥50%. Most recently, the FDA broadened approval for pembrolizumab in the first-line setting to include patients with stage III NSCLC and also

Table 1
Selected phase III data and regulatory approvals for anti-PD-1/PD-L1 in non-small cell lung cancer

Agent	FDA Approval	Study	Regimen	Survival Outcome	EMA Approval	PMDA Approval
PD-1						
Nivolumab	Second-line monotherapy non-squamous, metastatic	Borghaei et al,[20] 2015 (CheckMate-057, phase 3)	Nivolumab (3 mg/kg Q2 w) vs docetaxel	mOS: 12.2 vs 9.4 mo	Yes	Yes
	Second-line monotherapy, squamous, metastatic	Brahmer et al,[19] 2015 (CheckMate-017, phase 3)	Nivolumab (3 mg/kg Q2 w) vs docetaxel	mOS: 9.2 vs 6.0 mo	Yes	Yes
Pembrolizumab	First-line monotherapy, stage III/IV, TPS >1%	Mok et al,[6] 2019 (Keynote-042, phase 3)	Pembrolizumab (200 mg Q3 w) vs platinum chemo	mOS PD-L1 $\geq$50%: 20.0 vs 12.2 mo mOS PD-L1 $\geq$20%: 17.7 vs 13.0 mo mOS PD-L1 $\geq$1%: 16.7 vs 12.1 mo	Yes, metastatic, TPS >50%, no EGFR or ALK	Yes
	First-line combination non-squamous, metastatic	Gandhi et al,[68] 2018 (Keynote-189, phase 3)	Pembrolizumab (200 mg) + pemetrexed + carboplatin vs chemo	mOS: Not reached vs 11.3 mo	Yes	Yes
	First-line combination, squamous, metastatic	Paz-Ares et al,[39] 2018 (Keynote-407, phase 3)	Pembrolizumab (200 mg) + carboplatin + paclitaxel/ nab-paclitaxel vs chemo	mOS: 15.9 vs 11.3 mo	Yes	Yes
	Second-line monotherapy, metastatic, TPS >1%	Herbst et al,[23] 2016 (Keynote-010, phase 2/3)	Pembrolizumab 2 mg/kg vs pembrolizumab 10 mg/kg vs docetaxel	mOS: 10.4 vs 12.7 vs 8.5 mo		

PD-L1						
Atezolizumab	First-line combination, metastatic, no EGFR or ALK Second-line combination, metastatic	Socinski et al,[40] 2018 (IMPower 150, phase 3)	Atezolizumab + bevacizumab + carboplatin + paclitaxel (ABCP) vs ACP vs BCP	mOS: 19.2 vs not estimable vs 14.7 mo	Yes	Yes
	Second-line monotherapy, metastatic	Rittmeyer et al,[27] 2017 (OAK, phase 3)	Atezolizumab (1200 mg) vs docetaxel	mOS: 13.8 vs 9.6 mo		
Durvalumab	Maintenance monotherapy after chemoRT, stage III unresectable	Antonia et al,[30] 2018 (PACIFIC, phase 3)	Durvalumab (10 mg/kg) vs placebo	mOS: Not reached (33.3 mo median follow-up) vs 29.1 mo	Yes	Yes
CTLA-4 + PD-1						
Ipilimumab + nivolumab	Not yet approved	Hellmann et al,[35] 2019 (Checkmate-227, phase 3)	First line: nivolumab (3 mg/kg Q2 w) + ipilimumab (1 mg/kg Q6 w) vs nivolumab (240 mg Q2 w) vs chemo	mOS PD-L1 >1%: 17.1 vs 15.7 vs 14.9 mo mOS PD-L1 <1%: 17.2 vs 15.2 vs 12.2 mo		
Negative Studies						
PD-L1						
Avelumab		Barlesi et al,[69] 2018 (Javelin Lung, 200, phase 3)	Second line: avelumab (10 mg/kg) vs docetaxel	mOS: 11.4 vs 10.3 mo		

Abbreviations: mo, months; mOS, median overall survival; TPS, tumor proportion score; w, weeks.

lowered the PD-L1 cutoff to ≥1% based on results from Keynote-042. In this larger phase III trial comparing pembrolizumab (200 mg) versus platinum-based chemotherapy in patients with previously untreated advanced NSCLC (n = 1274) at various PD-L1 expression levels, median OS was significantly improved in all of the pembrolizumab groups (see **Table 1**).[6] These results confirmed efficacy of pembrolizumab monotherapy in patients with PD-L1 ≥50% and also demonstrated benefit in patients with the lower cutoff of PD-L1 ≥1%.

Atezolizumab

Atezolizumab is a humanized IgG1 monoclonal antibody against PD-L1 that was FDA approved for the treatment of patients with metastatic NSCLC in the second-line setting, based on positive results in large phase I,[25] phase II (POPLAR),[26] and phase III (OAK)[27] trials. The OAK trial was a large, randomized, international trial comparing atezolizumab (1200 mg) with docetaxel in patients with advanced NSCLC (n-1225), stratified by PD-L1 expression: PD-L1 ≥1%, PD-L1 ≥5%, and PD-L1 ≥50%. Median OS in the intention to treat population was statistically significantly greater in the atezolizumab group at 13.8 months (95% CI: 11.8–15.7) compared with 9.6 months in the docetaxel group (95% CI: 8.6–11.2). OS was improved with atezolizumab regardless of level of PD-L1 expression, with mOS in all PD-L1-positive patients treated with atezolizumab of 15.7 months (95% CI: 12.6–18.0) versus 10.3 months with docetaxel (95% CI: 8.8–12.0). PFS was similar for patients treated with atezolizumab (2.8 months) versus docetaxel (4.0 months), but median DOR was longer with atezolizumab (16.3 months) compared with docetaxel (6.2 months). There were more treatment-related AEs leading to discontinuation in the docetaxel group (19%) than in the atezolizumab group (8%).

Durvalumab

Durvalumab is a high-affinity, human IgG1 monoclonal antibody against PD-L1, which was first FDA approved for the treatment of previously treated locally advanced or metastatic urothelial carcinoma based on the interim analysis of a phase I/II trial demonstrating efficacy in the PD-L1-positive subgroup.[28] Following encouraging results in a phase I/II dose-escalation and expansion study,[29] durvalumab was evaluated in a randomized, international phase III trial (PACIFIC) as maintenance therapy after chemoradiotherapy for stage III, unresectable NSCLC.[5] Patients received either durvalumab 10 mg/kg as consolidation therapy for up to 12 months versus placebo (n = 709). The planned interim analysis met its primary endpoint of PFS: the median PFS from randomization was 16.8 months with durvalumab (95% CI: 13.0–18.1) versus 5.6 months with placebo. The 18-month PFS rate was 44.2% for durvalumab (95% CI: 37.7–50.5) compared with 27.0% with placebo, and this PFS benefit was irrespective of PD-L1 expression. AEs were similar in both groups, and grade 3 or 4 AEs were 29.9% with durvalumab compared with 26.1% with placebo. These results led to FDA approval of durvalumab as consolidation therapy, before reporting of the second primary endpoint of OS, which was impressive as median OS was not reached in the durvalumab group with 33.3 months median follow-up, compared with mOS 29.1 months in the placebo group.[30] Updated PFS was also reported, with median PFS with durvalumab 17.2 months (95% CI: 13.1–23.9) versus 5.6 months (95% CI: 4.6–7.7) with placebo. The safety profile was similar, and again noted was the higher rate of pneumonitis with durvalumab compared with placebo. This was further explored, and both Asian patients (47.9% vs 17.6%) and patients with EGFR mutations (11.0% vs 3.8%) were more likely to have AE pneumonitis.[31]

CLINICAL DATA OF IMMUNE CHECKPOINT COMBINATION THERAPY IN NON-SMALL CELL LUNG CANCER: DUAL IMMUNOTHERAPY

Ipilimumab Plus Nivolumab

Ipilimumab is a fully human anti-CTLA-4 that was first approved by the FDA as monotherapy for previously treated metastatic melanoma based on phase III data.[13] The combination of ipilimumab and nivolumab was then evaluated in untreated melanoma in a phase I trial evaluating both sequential and concurrent treatment.[32] Positive results in the ensuing phase II trial comparing the combination of ipilimumab plus nivolumab versus ipilimumab monotherapy[33] led to FDA approval of the combination for the treatment of unresectable or metastatic melanoma. Given the evidence in favor of combination immunotherapy for melanoma, the combination of ipilimumab plus nivolumab was evaluated in NSCLC in a phase 1 multicohort study (CheckMate-012).[34] Patients were randomized to 3 different dosing/scheduling regimens: nivolumab 1 mg/kg every 2 weeks plus ipilimumab 1 mg/kg every 6 weeks, nivolumab 3 mg/kg every 2 weeks plus ipilimumab 1 mg/kg every 12 weeks, and nivolumab 3 mg/g every 2 weeks plus ipilimumab 1 mg/kg every 6 weeks, with results reported for the nivolumab 3 mg/kg doses. Safety endpoints were met with treatment-related serious AEs in 32% of the patients in the ipilimumab every 12 weeks group, and 28% of the patients in the ipilimumab every 6 weeks group. Confirmed objective responses were seen in 47% of patients treated with the ipilimumab every 12 weeks, and in 38% of the patients treated with ipilimumab every 6 weeks. This was further improved in patients with PD-L1 expression ≥1% to 57% with objective responses in both cohorts. Median PFS in the PD-L1-positive patients treated with ipilimumab every 12 weeks was 8.1 months (95% CI: 5.6–not reached), and 10.6 months (95% CI: 3.5–not reached) in those treated with ipilimumab every 6 weeks.

With these promising results, a large, randomized phase III trial (CheckMate-227) was done to further evaluate the clinical benefit of the combination of nivolumab plus ipilimumab in patients with advanced, previously untreated NSCLC (n = 1739).[35] This 2-part trial randomized patients with PD-L1 ≥1% in part 1a to receive nivolumab plus ipilimumab, nivolumab alone, or platinum-doublet chemotherapy; patients with PD-L1 ≤1% in part 1b received nivolumab plus ipilimumab, nivolumab plus platinum-doublet chemotherapy, or platinum-doublet chemotherapy. The most notable results were in the comparison of patients treated with nivolumab plus ipilimumab compared with chemotherapy. In patients with PD-L1 ≥1%, median OS was 17.1 months (95% CI: 15.0–20.1) with nivolumab plus ipilimumab, compared with 14.9 months with chemotherapy alone (P=.007), and the HR for death was 0.79 (97.72% CI: 0.65–0.96). More significantly, the median DOR was 23.2 months in the combination immunotherapy group versus 6.2 months in the chemotherapy group, and patients with an ongoing response at 2 years was 49.5% in the combination group versus 11.0% in the chemotherapy group. Median OS was also significantly improved in patients with PD-L1 ≤1% who received combination therapy (17.2 months, 95% CI: 12.8–22.0) compared with chemotherapy (12.2 months), with HR for death 0.62 (95% CI: 0.48–0.78). Benefit was also seen in PFS, ORR, and DOR regardless of PD-L1 expression. Although combination immunotherapy is not yet approved for the treatment of NSCLC, it is likely that it will soon be another FDA-approved indication, potentially regardless of PD-L1 expression.

An earlier phase II trial, CheckMate-568, evaluated the combination of nivolumab plus ipilimumab based on tumor mutational burden (TMB), the number of mutations in cancer cells. As it demonstrated improved response and PFS in patients with TMB ≥ 10 mutations/megabase (mut/Mb),[36] PFS in patients with TMB ≥ 10 mut/Mb regardless of PD-L1 expression was also separately analyzed as a coprimary endpoint in CheckMate-227.[37] Results were promising, with median PFS in the high TMB group 7.2 months with nivolumab plus ipilimumab (95% CI: 5.5–13.2) versus 5.5 months with chemotherapy, and response rate of 45.3% with nivolumab plus ipilimumab compared with 26.9% with chemotherapy. However, the OS was similar regardless of TMB and when combining PD-L1 expression and TMB.[35] There remains no predictive biomarker of response for ICIs, which will be further discussed below (see Future Directions).

CLINICAL DATA OF IMMUNE CHECKPOINT COMBINATION THERAPY IN NON-SMALL CELL LUNG CANCER: IMMUNOTHERAPY/CHEMOTHERAPY COMBINATIONS

Pembrolizumab Plus Chemotherapy

With the success of pembrolizumab as a monotherapy and more understanding of the antitumor mechanism of chemotherapy, evaluating for synergy in the combination of ICI with chemotherapy seemed like a natural next step. The addition of pembrolizumab to the platinum doublet of carboplatin and pemetrexed was first evaluated in a randomized, phase II study (Keynote-021) in patients with untreated, advanced, non-squamous NSCLC (n = 123).[38] A significantly higher proportion of patients treated with pembrolizumab plus chemotherapy (55%, 95% CI: 42–68) had an objective response compared with the chemotherapy-only group (29%, 95% CI: 18–41). The secondary endpoint of PFS was significantly higher for patients treated with pembrolizumab plus chemotherapy (mPFS 13.0 months, 95% CI: 8.3–not reached) compared with chemotherapy alone (mPFS 8.9 months). These results led to accelerated FDA approval of the combination of pembrolizumab with pemetrexed and platinum as first-line therapy for metastatic, non-squamous NSCLC. Results from the ensuing phase III study (Keynote-189) led to regular approval the following year. Keynote-189 compared pembrolizumab plus chemotherapy or placebo plus chemotherapy in 616 patients with metastatic, untreated, non-squamous NSCLC. Both primary endpoints of OS and PFS were met, with median OS not reached in the pembrolizumab plus chemotherapy group and 11.3 months in the placebo-chemotherapy group. The HR for death was 0.49 (95% CI: 0.38–0.64). Median PFS was 8.8 months (95% CI: 7.6–9.2) in the pembrolizumab plus chemotherapy group compared with 4.9 months in the placebo-combination group. This combination regimen now constitutes a new standard of care for newly diagnosed patients with advanced non-squamous NSCLC, regardless of PD-L1 expression. The question of whether to use pembrolizumab monotherapy or the combination with chemotherapy for high PD-L1 expressors (>50%) is an open question.

Pembrolizumab in combination with chemotherapy was also evaluated in patients with untreated, metastatic, squamous NSCLC (n = 559) in the phase III Keynote-407 trial.[39] Patients were stratified by PD-L1 expression, and the trial had 2 primary endpoints of OS and PFS, both of which were met. The median OS in the pembrolizumab plus chemotherapy group was 15.9 months (95% CI: 13.2–not reached) compared with 11.3 months in the placebo plus chemotherapy group. Benefit was seen regardless of PD-L1 expression for OS and also for PFS, with incremental improvement with increasing PD-L1 expression. The median PFS for the pembrolizumab plus chemotherapy group was 6.4 months (95% CI: 6.2–8.3) compared with 4.8 months for the placebo plus chemotherapy group. The rate of AEs was similar in both groups. The results of this trial led to FDA approval of pembrolizumab plus chemotherapy for metastatic squamous NSCLC. This is also a new recent standard of care for patients with metastatic squamous NSCLC, regardless of PD-L1 expression, with similar questions relating to choice of monotherapy versus combination in high expressors of PD-L1.

Atezolizumab Plus Chemotherapy Plus Bevacizumab

Yet another combination strategy that was recently evaluated in patients with metastatic NSCLC was the combination of atezolizumab with bevacizumab, an inhibitor of vascular endothelial growth factor was studied in the IMpower150 study.[40,41] IMpower150 was a large, randomized trial of patients with metastatic non-squamous NSCLC (n = 1045) comparing atezolizumab plus bevacizumab plus chemotherapy (ABCP) versus atezolizumab plus chemotherapy (ACP) versus bevacizumab plus chemotherapy (BCP). Due to improvement in OS and PFS with ABCP (mOS 19.2 months, mPFS 8.3 months) compared with BCP (mOS 14.7 months, mPFS 6.8 months) regardless of PD-L1 expression and EGFR or ALK gene alteration status, the 4-drug regimen received FDA approval. This also represents a first-line treatment option for patients with newly diagnosed stage IV NSCLC regardless of PD-L1 expression.

FUTURE DIRECTIONS

Biomarkers of Response

Although ICIs have transformed outcomes for patients with many other types of cancer, most NSCLC patients' cancers will ultimately progress, and some patient's NSCLCs will not respond to immunotherapy. This is true across tumor types, and there is currently no biomarker that has been validated across tumor types to predict response to therapy. PD-L1 expression, tested by IHC, is currently the only validated biomarker, and FDA approvals for some ICIs in several cancers, including bladder cancer, NSCLC, triple-negative breast cancer, cervical cancer, and gastric cancer are linked to PD-L1 status.[42] There are currently 5 PD-L1 assays with FDA approval, each developed for a different ICI: PD-L1 IHC 22C3 pharmDx as a companion diagnostic for pembrolizumab, PD-L1 IHC 28 to 8 pharmDx as a complementary diagnostic for nivolumab, VENTANA PD-L1 (SP142) assay as a complementary diagnostic for atezolizumab, VENTANA PD-L1 (SP263) assay as a complementary diagnostic for durvalumab (bladder cancer only), and most recently PD-L1 IHC 73-10 assay for avelumab. The multitude of assays antibodies and different scoring systems complicates the use of PD-L1 expression in clinical practice. The Blueprint PD-L1 Assay IHC Comparison Project initially compared the first 4 assays and cutoffs, and found that the 22C3, 28-8, and SP263 assays were interchangeable, and the SP142 assay less sensitive than the others.[43] Phase 2 of the Blueprint study also analyzed the 73-10 assay, and found it to have greater sensitivity than the other 4 assays.[44] Phase 2B of the Blueprint study compared samples of tumor resection, small biopsy, and needle aspirate of the same tumor and found no significant difference on PD-L1 scoring among them, although scoring was not possible in 14% of the aspirates.[45] This issue of obtaining samples for PD-L1 testing is potentially magnified in NSCLC, as cytology is a common way of diagnosing NSCLC. In addition, PD-L1 expression is heterogeneous, with low interobserver reproducibility.[46] Although PD-L1 expression is actively used in the clinic to determine eligibility for treatment of patients with NSCLC with pembrolizumab, methods to standardize PD-L1 evaluation are ongoing.

TMB is another potential marker that has shown particular promise in NSCLC but needs to be validated prospectively.[47,48] Somatic mutations in the DNA of affected cells accumulate over time and ultimately cause neoplastic transformation. Some of these mutations generate neoantigens, which can be recognized by the immune system, and TMB can be used to estimate the tumor neoantigen load.[49] Higher numbers of mutations was first found to be associated with improved response and PFS in patients with NSCLC treated with pembrolizumab retrospectively,.[50] This led to the evaluation of TMB as a potential biomarker of response in relation to other anti-PD-1/PD-L1 ICIs. In CheckMate-026, a phase III trial of nivolumab monotherapy versus chemotherapy in patients with metastatic NSCLC with PD-L1 $\geq$1%, patients with high TMB (defined as $\geq$243 missense mutations, or the upper tertile) were found to have a higher response rate (47% vs 28%) and PFS (9.7 vs 5.8 months).[51] Blood-based TMB (bTMB) has also been evaluated prospectively. In the B-F1RST study, a trial of atezolizumab monotherapy in patients with untreated stage III/IV NSCLC, patients with high bTMB, defined as $\geq$16 mut/Mb, had improved PFS and OS with atezolizumab.[52] However, there are also severl assays for TMB, and no standardized cutoff for high TMB. In addition, the number of mutations in different tumor types is highly variable,[53] particularly in NSCLC, as there are more mutations in the tumors of smokers than never-smokers,[54] and not all mutations result in a neoantigen or functional T cell response. Identification of further predictive biomarkers of response to anti-PD-1/PD-L1 remains an area of active research in NSCLC and other tumor types.

The Gut Microbiome

The gut microbiome is another emerging biomarker of response that is uniquely a modifiable feature of the host, whereas TMB and PD-L1 are nonmodifiable features of the tumor. The microbiome is the population of microorganisms in a specific biological environment, and the gut microbiome has been implicated as one of the determinants for the efficacy of ICIs.[55] The gut microbiome refers to the collective genomes of the microorganisms that reside in the digestive tract, and next-generation sequencing has allowed for culture-independent cataloging of entire genomes of individual organisms' microbiomes.[56,57] The gut microbiome was first shown to be implicated in response to ICIs in patients with metastatic melanoma treated with ipilimumab, evaluated through fecal microbiota transfer to antibiotic-treated mouse models.[58] Specific strains of *Bacteroides* (*B fragilis* and/or *B thetaiotaomicron*) and *Burkholderiales cepacia* in the gut were associated with improved anti-cancer responses. The first prospective study in humans evaluating the gut microbiota and its effect on response to ICIs was also done in metastatic melanoma, and found improved PFS and OS in patients whose microbiota was enriched with *Faecalibacterium* and other Firmicutes.[59] This led to further research in melanoma, as well as in other tumors, including NSCLC. In a cohort of patients with NSCLC (n = 60) and renal cell carcinoma (n = 40), patients whose gut microbiome had greater numbers of microbial species (termed alpha-diversity), and the presence of *Akkermansia mucinphila*, there was an association with improved responses to ICIs. Interestingly, these data and others have observed that antibiotic use may be implicated in lack of response to ICIs,[60] There is variation in specific bacterial taxa, which have demonstrated an association with response to ICIs in different studies, and this may potentially be due to different sequencing techniques. Importantly, there is currently no standardized approach to microbiome analysis.[61] There is still much to be understood in the role of the microbiome in patients treated with ICIs, including continued identification of bacteria and metabolites as well as the actual mechanisms of the microbiome's immunologic impact.

Neoadjuvant Immune Checkpoint Inhibitors in Non-small Cell Lung Cancer

Neoadjuvant ICI has shown promise in other solid tumors, such as melanoma[62] and breast cancer.[63] A mouse model of triple-negative breast cancer demonstrated improved survival in mice treated with neoadjuvant therapy compared with adjuvant therapy, and these mice also had an increase in tumor-specific T cells.[64] A pilot study of neoadjuvant nivolumab for resectable NSCLC (n = 21) showed promising results, with no delays in surgery and a major pathologic response in 45% of patients.[65] In addition, tumors with a major pathologic response had a higher frequency of T cell clones that had expanded in peripheral blood after PD-1 blockade. Neoadjuvant nivolumab is now being evaluated in a larger clinical trial. Of note, the availability of posttreatment resection specimens also allowed for in-depth histologic analysis, leading to a proposal for a standardized "Immune-Related Pathologic Response Criteria", which was also demonstrated to be reproducible between pathologists.[66] These criteria are now being used in other trials of neoadjuvant ICIs in NSCLC. The success with nivolumab sparked a neoadjuvant trial with atezolizumab for resectable NSCLC, with results of the initial safety analysis (n = 21) without major delays in surgery, and neoadjuvant atezolizumab was well tolerated.[67] If results continue to be promising, it is likely that there will be a role for neoadjuvant ICI in the treatment of resectable NSCLC.

SUMMARY

Immunotherapy in the form of anti-PD-1/PD-L1 ICIs has transformed the treatment of NSCLC and survival in a subset of patients with advanced NSCLC. Several ICIs have FDA approval in stage III NSCLC, stage IV NSCLC, and now both as monotherapy and in combination with chemotherapy or a second immunotherapy agent. Using ICIs in the neoadjuvant setting has allowed for more understanding of the antitumor response, and additional investigation of potential predictive biomarkers of response, such as the gut microbiome is likely to uncover a deeper understanding of the mechanisms of ICIs.

DISCLOSURE

M.L. Hsu: Nothing to disclose. J. Naidoo: Research funding: Merck (United States), AstraZeneca (United States); Consulting: AstraZeneca, Bristol-Myers Squibb, Roche/Genentech; Honoraria: AstraZeneca, Bristol-Myers Squibb.

REFERENCES

1. Sharma P, Allison JP. The future of immune checkpoint therapy. Science 2015;348(6230):56–61.
2. Pardoll DM. The blockade of immune checkpoints in cancer immunotherapy. Nat Rev Cancer 2012. https://doi.org/10.1038/nrc3239.
3. FDA Approved Drug Products, Ipilimumab.. Available at: https://www.accessdata.fda.gov/scripts/cder/daf/index.cfm?event=overview.process&ApplNo=125377. Accessed November 14, 2019.
4. Darvin P, Toor SM, Sasidharan Nair V, et al. Immune checkpoint inhibitors: recent progress and potential biomarkers. Exp Mol Med 2018;50(12). https://doi.org/10.1038/s12276-018-0191-1.
5. Antonia SJ, Villegas A, Daniel D, et al. Durvalumab after chemoradiotherapy in stage III non-small-cell lung cancer. N Engl J Med 2017;377(20):1919–29.
6. Mok TSK, Wu YL, Kudaba I, et al. Pembrolizumab versus chemotherapy for previously untreated, PD-L1-expressing, locally advanced or metastatic non-small-cell lung cancer (KEYNOTE-042): a randomised, open-label, controlled, phase 3 trial. Lancet 2019;393(10183):1819–30.
7. FDA grants regular approval for pembrolizumab in combination with chemotherapy for first-line treatment of metastatic nonsquamous NSCLC. 2018. Available at: https://www.fda.gov/drugs/resources-information-approved-drugs/fda-grants-regular-approval-pembrolizumab-combination-chemotherapy-first-line-treatment-metastatic. Accessed November 14, 2019.
8. Kazandjian D, Suzman DL, Blumenthal G, et al. FDA approval summary: nivolumab for the treatment of metastatic non-small cell lung cancer with progression on or after platinum-based chemotherapy. Oncologist 2016;21(5):634–42.
9. FDA approves atezolizumab with chemotherapy and bevacizumab for first-line treatment of metastatic non-squamous NSCLC. 2018. Available at: https://www.fda.gov/drugs/fda-approves-atezolizumab-chemotherapy-and-bevacizumab-first-line-treatment-metastatic-non-squamous. Accessed November 14, 2019.
10. Leach DR, Krummel MF, Allison JP. Enhancement of antitumor immunity by CTLA-4 blockade. Science 1996;271:1734–6.
11. Krummel MF, Allison JP. CTLA-4 engagement inhibits IL-2 accumulation and cell cycle progression upon activation of resting T cells. J Exp Med 1996;183(6):2533–40.
12. Hurwitz AA, Yu TFY, Leach DR, et al. CTLA-4 blockade synergizes with tumor-derived granulocyte-macrophage colony-stimulating factor for treatment of an experimental mammary carcinoma. Proc Natl Acad Sci U S A 1998;95(17):10067–71.
13. Stephen Hodi F, O'Day SJ, McDermott DF, et al. Improved survival with ipilimumab in patients with metastatic melanoma. N Engl J Med 2010;8:711–34.
14. Parry RV, Chemnitz JM, Frauwirth KA, et al. CTLA-4 and PD-1 receptors inhibit T-cell activation by distinct mechanisms. Mol Cell Biol 2005;25(21):9543–53.
15. Agata Y, Kawasaki A, Nishimura H, et al. Expression of the PD-1 antigen on the surface of stimulated mouse T and B lymphocytes, 8, 1996. Available at: https://academic.oup.com/intimm/article-abstract/8/5/765/693918. Accessed November 23, 2019.
16. Freeman GJ, Long AJ, Iwai Y, et al. Engagement of the PD-1 immunoinhibitory receptor by a novel B7 family member leads to negative regulation of lymphocyte activation. J Exp Med 2000;192(7):1027–34.
17. Dong H, Strome SE, Salomao DR, et al. Tumor-associated B7-H1 promotes T-cell apoptosis: a potential mechanism of immune evasion. Nat Med 2002;8(8):793–800.
18. Topalian SL, Drake CG, Pardoll DM. Targeting the PD-1/B7-H1(PD-L1) pathway to activate anti-tumor immunity. Curr Opin Immunol 2012;24(2):207–12.
19. Brahmer J, Reckamp KL, Baas P, et al. Nivolumab versus docetaxel in advanced squamous-cell non-small-cell lung cancer. N Engl J Med 2015;373(2):123–35.
20. Borghaei H, Paz-Ares L, Horn L, et al. Nivolumab versus docetaxel in advanced nonsquamous non-small-cell lung cancer. N Engl J Med 2015;373(17):1627–39.
21. Hamid O, Robert C, Daud A, et al. Safety and tumor responses with lambrolizumab (anti–PD-1) in melanoma. N Engl J Med 2013;369(2):134–44.

22. Garon EB, Rizvi NA, Hui R, et al. Pembrolizumab for the treatment of non-small-cell lung cancer. N Engl J Med 2015;372(21):2018–28.
23. Herbst RS, Baas P, Kim DW, et al. Pembrolizumab versus docetaxel for previously treated, PD-L1-positive, advanced non-small-cell lung cancer (KEYNOTE-010): a randomised controlled trial. Lancet 2016;387(10027):1540–50.
24. Reck M, Rodriguez-Abreu D, Robinson AG, et al. Pembrolizumab versus chemotherapy for PD-L1-positive non-small-cell lung cancer. N Engl J Med 2016;375(19):1823–33.
25. Herbst RS, Soria JC, Kowanetz M, et al. Predictive correlates of response to the anti-PD-L1 antibody MPDL3280A in cancer patients. Nature 2014; 515(7528):563–7.
26. Fehrenbacher L, Spira A, Ballinger M, et al. Atezolizumab versus docetaxel for patients with previously treated non-small-cell lung cancer (POPLAR): a multicentre, open-label, phase 2 randomised controlled trial. Lancet 2016;387(10030):1837–46.
27. Rittmeyer A, Barlesi F, Waterkamp D, et al. Atezolizumab versus docetaxel in patients with previously treated non-small-cell lung cancer (OAK): a phase 3, open-label, multicentre randomised controlled trial. Lancet 2017;389(10066):255–65.
28. Massard C, Gordon MS, Sharma S, et al. Safety and efficacy of durvalumab (MEDI4736), an anti-programmed cell death ligand-1 immune checkpoint inhibitor, in patients with advanced urothelial bladder cancer. J Clin Oncol 2016;34(26): 3119–25.
29. Antonia SJ, Brahmer JR, Balmanoukian AS, et al. Safety and clinical activity of first-line durvalumab in advanced NSCLC: Updated results from a phase 1/2 study. J Clin Oncol 2017;35(15_suppl): e20504.
30. Antonia SJ, Villegas A, Daniel D, et al. Overall survival with durvalumab after chemoradiotherapy in stage III NSCLC. N Engl J Med 2018;379(24): 2342–50.
31. Vansteenkiste J, Naidoo J, Faivre-Finn C, et al. MA05.02 PACIFIC subgroup analysis: pneumonitis in stage III, unresectable NSCLC patients treated with durvalumab vs. placebo after CRT. J Thorac Oncol 2018;13(10):S370–1.
32. Wolchok JD, Kluger H, Callahan MK, et al. Nivolumab plus ipilimumab in advanced melanoma. N Engl J Med 2013;369(2):122–33.
33. Postow MA, Chesney J, Pavlick AC, et al. Nivolumab and ipilimumab versus ipilimumab in untreated melanoma. N Engl J Med 2015;372(21):2006–17.
34. Hellmann MD, Rizvi NA, Goldman JW, et al. Nivolumab plus ipilimumab as first-line treatment for advanced non-small-cell lung cancer (CheckMate 012): results of an open-label, phase 1, multicohort study. Lancet Oncol 2017;18(1):31–41.
35. Hellmann MD, Paz-Ares L, Bernabe Caro R, et al. Nivolumab plus ipilimumab in advanced non-small-cell lung cancer. N Engl J Med 2019. https://doi.org/10.1056/NEJMoa1910231. NEJMoa1910231.
36. Ready N, Hellmann MD, Awad MM, et al. First-line nivolumab plus ipilimumab in advanced non-small-cell lung cancer (CheckMate 568): Outcomes by programmed death ligand 1 and tumor mutational burden as biomarkers. J Clin Oncol 2019;37: 992–1000.
37. Hellmann MD, Ciuleanu T-E, Pluzanski A, et al. Nivolumab plus ipilimumab in lung cancer with a high tumor mutational burden. N Engl J Med 2018;378(22): 2093–104.
38. Langer CJ, Gadgeel SM, Borghaei H, et al. Carboplatin and pemetrexed with or without pembrolizumab for advanced, non-squamous non-small-cell lung cancer: a randomised, phase 2 cohort of the open-label KEYNOTE-021 study. Lancet Oncol 2016;17(11):1497–508.
39. Paz-Ares L, Luft A, Vicente D, et al. Pembrolizumab plus chemotherapy for squamous non-small-cell lung cancer. N Engl J Med 2018;379(21):2040–51.
40. Socinski MA, Jotte RM, Cappuzzo F, et al. Atezolizumab for first-line treatment of metastatic nonsquamous NSCLC. N Engl J Med 2018;378(24): 2288–301.
41. Hegde PS, Wallin JJ, Mancao C. Predictive markers of anti-VEGF and emerging role of angiogenesis inhibitors as immunotherapeutics. Semin Cancer Biol 2018;52:117–24.
42. Davis AA, Patel VG. The role of PD-L1 expression as a predictive biomarker: an analysis of all US Food and Drug Administration (FDA) approvals of immune checkpoint inhibitors. J Immunother Cancer 2019; 7(1):278.
43. Hirsch FR, McElhinny A, Stanforth D, et al. PD-L1 immunohistochemistry assays for lung cancer: results from phase 1 of the blueprint Pd-L1 IHC assay comparison project. J Thorac Oncol 2017;12(2): 208–22.
44. Tsao MS, Kerr KM, Kockx M, et al. PD-L1 immunohistochemistry comparability study in real-life clinical samples: results of blueprint phase 2 project. J Thorac Oncol 2018;13(9):1302–11.
45. Kerr K, Tsao M, Yatabe Y, et al. OA03.03 phase 2B of blueprint PD-L1 immunohistochemistry assay comparability study. J Thorac Oncol 2018;13(10): S325.
46. McLaughlin J, Han G, Schalper KA, et al. Quantitative assessment of the heterogeneity of PD-L1 expression in non-small-cell lung cancer. JAMA Oncol 2016;2(1):46–54.
47. Greillier L, Tomasini P, Barlesi F. The clinical utility of tumor mutational burden in non-small cell lung cancer. Transl Lung Cancer Res 2018;7(6): 639–46.

48. Chan TA, Yarchoan M, Jaffee E, et al. Development of tumor mutation burden as an immunotherapy biomarker: utility for the oncology clinic. Ann Oncol 2019;30(1):44–56.
49. Campesato LF, Barroso-Sousa R, Jimenez L, et al. Comprehensive cancer-gene panels can be used to estimate mutational load and predict clinical benefit to PD-1 blockade in clinical practice. Oncotarget 2015;6(33):34221–7.
50. Rizvi NA, Hellmann MD, Snyder A, et al. Mutational landscape determines sensitivity to PD-1 blockade in non-small cell lung cancer. Science 2015; 348(6230):124–8.
51. Carbone DP, Reck M, Paz-Ares L, et al. First-line nivolumab in stage IV or recurrent non–small-cell lung cancer. N Engl J Med 2017;376(25):2415–26.
52. Socinski M, Velcheti V, Mekhail T, et al. LBA83Final efficacy results from B-F1RST, a prospective phase II trial evaluating blood-based tumour mutational burden (bTMB) as a predictive biomarker for atezolizumab (atezo) in 1L non-small cell lung cancer (NSCLC). Ann Oncol 2019;30(Supplement_5). https://doi.org/10.1093/annonc/mdz394.081.
53. Lawrence MS, Stojanov P, Polak P, et al. Mutational heterogeneity in cancer and the search for new cancer-associated genes. Nature 2013;499(7457): 214–8.
54. Govindan R, Ding L, Griffith M, et al. Genomic landscape of non-small cell lung cancer in smokers and never-smokers. Cell 2012;150(6):1121–34.
55. Lynch SV, Pedersen O. The human intestinal microbiome in health and disease. N Engl J Med 2016; 375(24):2369–79.
56. Qin J, Li R, Raes J, et al. A human gut microbial gene catalog established by metagenomic sequencing. Nature 2010;464(7285):59–65.
57. Zitvogel L, Galluzzi L, Viaud S, et al. Cancer and the gut microbiota: an unexpected link. Sci Transl Med 2015;7(271). https://doi.org/10.1126/scitranslmed.3010473.
58. Vétizou M, Pitt JM, Daillère R, et al. Anticancer immunotherapy by CTLA-4 blockade relies on the gut microbiota. Science 2015;350(6264):1079–84.
59. Chaput N, Lepage P, Coutzac C, et al. Baseline gut microbiota predicts clinical response and colitis in metastatic melanoma patients treated with ipilimumab. Ann Oncol 2017;28(6):1368–79.
60. Routy B, Le Chatelier E, Derosa L, et al. Gut microbiome influences efficacy of PD-1-based immunotherapy against epithelial tumors. Science 2018; 359(6371):91–7.
61. Gopalakrishnan V, Helmink BA, Spencer CN, et al. The influence of the gut microbiome on cancer, immunity, and cancer immunotherapy. Cancer Cell 2018;33(4):570–80.
62. Rozeman EA, Van Akkooi ACJ, Menzies AM, et al. Multicenter phase 2 study to identify the optimal neo-adjuvant combination scheme of ipilimumab (IPI) and nivolumab (NIVO) (OpACIN-neo). J Clin Oncol 2018;36(15_suppl):TPS9606.
63. Schmid P, Park YH, Muñoz-Couselo E, et al. Pembrolizumab (pembro) + chemotherapy (chemo) as neoadjuvant treatment for triple negative breast cancer (TNBC): preliminary results from KEYNOTE-173. J Clin Oncol 2017;35(15_suppl):556.
64. Liu J, Blake SJ, Yong MCR, et al. Improved efficacy of neoadjuvant compared to adjuvant immunotherapy to eradicate metastatic disease. Cancer Discov 2016;6(12):1382–99.
65. Forde PM, Chaft JE, Smith KN, et al. Neoadjuvant PD-1 blockade in resectable lung cancer. N Engl J Med 2018;378(21):1976–86.
66. Cottrell TR, Thompson ED, Forde PM, et al. Pathologic features of response to neoadjuvant anti-PD-1 in resected non-small-cell lung carcinoma: a proposal for quantitative immune-related pathologic response criteria (irPRC). Ann Oncol 2018;29(8): 1853–60.
67. Rusch VW, Chaft JE, Johnson B, et al. Neoadjuvant atezolizumab in resectable non-small cell lung cancer (NSCLC): Initial results from a multicenter study (LCMC3). J Clin Oncol 2018;36(15_suppl):8541.
68. Gandhi L, Rodríguez-Abreu D, Gadgeel S, et al. Pembrolizumab plus chemotherapy in metastatic non-small-cell lung cancer. N Engl J Med 2018; 378(22):2078–92.
69. Barlesi F, Vansteenkiste J, Spigel D, et al. Avelumab versus docetaxel in patients with platinum-treated advanced non-small-cell lung cancer (JAVELIN Lung 200): an open-label, randomised, phase 3 study. Lancet Oncol 2018;19(11):1468–79.

Combining Immunotherapy and Chemotherapy for Non–Small Cell Lung Cancer

Julia Judd, DO, Hossein Borghaei, DO, MS*

KEYWORDS

• Non–small cell lung cancer • Adenocarcinoma • Squamous cell carcinoma
• Chemo-immunotherapy • Immunotherapy • Checkpoint inhibition • PD-1 inhibitor

KEY POINTS

- Adaptive immunity plays a major role in the prevention of tumor growth and development.
- Platinum-based chemotherapy augments antitumor immunity by inducing immunogenic cell death, increasing tumor neo-antigen expression, and disturbing the immunosuppressive tumor microenvironment that prevents immune detection.
- Antibodies targeting the PD-1 receptor-ligand interaction, which tumor cells exploit to evade immune detection, enhance the antitumor immune response.
- Based on preclinical studies, there is a strong rationale for combining platinum-based chemotherapy and immunotherapy and this potential synergistic effect has been verified with improved outcomes in the clinical setting.

INTRODUCTION: OVERVIEW OF ADVANCED NON–SMALL CELL LUNG CANCER TREATMENT

Lung cancer remains the leading cause of cancer-related deaths worldwide.[1] In the United States, there were an estimated 234,030 new lung cancer cases and 154,050 lung cancer–related deaths in 2018, with higher incidence and mortality in men compared with women. Non–small cell lung cancer (NSCLC) is the most common histologic subtype, accounting for approximately 85% of all lung cancer cases.[2] Unfortunately, most patients with lung cancer are deemed incurable, with advanced disease at diagnosis. Therefore, systemic therapy is the primary treatment option. Although pembrolizumab monotherapy has replaced cytotoxic chemotherapy as first-line treatment in patients whose tumor cell programmed death ligand 1 (PD-L1) staining (tumor proportion score) is ≥50%, this is only a fraction of patients with NSCLC.[3] It is important to maximize the response to first-line treatment, as more than half of patients with NSCLC clinically decline before ever receiving second-line therapy.[4] With many preclinical studies demonstrating immunomodulatory effects of cytotoxic chemotherapy, first-line clinical trials using combination therapy, with PD-1 receptor or ligand inhibitors and chemotherapy, were initiated to improve treatment response and prolong survival.[5–13] Recently, combination therapy has become the standard of care for most patients with NSCLC.

NON–SMALL CELL LUNG CANCER IMMUNOLOGY AND THE USE OF CHECKPOINT INHIBITION

Cancer is associated with a state of chronic inflammation, as well as severe systemic immune suppression.[14] Cancer develops by accumulating genetic alterations and the loss of normal cellular regulation. These events lead to the expression of neo-antigens, a peptide bound to major histocompatibility class I (MHC-I) molecules, on the cancer cell surface, which differentiates them

Department of Hematology/Oncology, Fox Chase Cancer Center, 333 Cottman Avenue, Philadelphia, PA 19111, USA
* Corresponding author.
E-mail address: Hossein.Borghaei@fccc.edu

Thorac Surg Clin 30 (2020) 199–206
https://doi.org/10.1016/j.thorsurg.2020.01.006

from normal cells.[15] It is well established that evasion of immune surveillance is one of the hallmarks of cancer.[16] Previously, development of new therapies had focused on direct tumor cytotoxicity and disturbing tumor microenvironment interactions, such as angiogenesis. However, ongoing research has determined that adaptive immunity plays a major role in the prevention of cancer growth.

The adaptive immune system can effectively kill cancer cells if a series of steps are able to occur. Initially, neo-antigens from the tumor cells are released and captured for processing by dendritic cells (DCs). Then the DCs present the tumor-specific antigens on MHC-I and MHC-II molecules to CD8+ and CD4+ T cells, respectively. This results in priming and activation of the effector T cells against the foreign antigen. At this stage, the ratio of T effector cells to regulatory T cells, which act by suppressing the immune response, determine the final outcome. The effector T cells will travel to the tumor and the T-cell receptor will recognize the tumor-specific antigen presented on the MHC-I complex on the tumor surface, resulting in destruction of the target cell. Subsequently, more tumor-associated antigens are released, thus enhancing tumor-specific immunity.[15] However, this cycle does not function properly in patients with cancer for a variety of reasons; tumor antigens may not be detected and captured by DCs, the antigens may be recognized as self and thus create a T regulatory response leading to tumor tolerance, T cells may not travel to or are prevented from infiltrating the tumors, and, importantly, the tumor microenvironment may suppress the effector cells from functioning.[15]

There are additional co-stimulatory receptors that regulate T-cell activation, also called immune-checkpoints. Under normal physiologic conditions, these molecules allow self-tolerance, but cancer cells exploit these molecules for immune evasion.[17] The PD-1 receptor on T cells interacts with the PD-L1/PD2 ligand (PD-L2) on antigen-presenting cells and peripheral tissue acting as a co-inhibitory signal to maintain self-tolerance. Following T-cell activation, the PD-1 receptor is expressed on T cells; however, concurrent activation of the ligand on macrophages and in tumor tissue prevents immune destruction. This interaction is manipulated by tumor cells to evade immune eradication and has become an important therapeutic target. Antibodies targeting PD-1 and PDL-1 have been developed that prevent this receptor-ligand interaction and, therefore, enhance the antitumor immune response.[18,19]

PLATINUM-BASED CHEMOTHERAPY IMMUNOMODULATION AND SYNERGY WITH IMMUNOTHERAPY

Platinum-based chemotherapy augments antitumor immunity by inducing immunogenic cell death (ICD), increasing tumor neo-antigen expression and also by disturbing the immunosuppressive tumor microenvironment that prevents immune detection.[6] ICD involves changes on the cell membrane that signal DCs to remove the dying cell followed by release of factors, which stimulates DC activation and maturation. Subsequently, DCs present tumor antigens to T cells creating tumor-specific effector cells.[6] Chemotherapy also alters the tumor microenvironment by promoting increased infiltration of CD8+ T cells, decreasing regulatory T cells and myeloid suppressor cells, and stimulating antigen-presenting cell maturation.[5,7,8] Several preclinical studies have demonstrated how chemotherapy can augment effector T-cell function by a variety of mechanisms. A study in mice treated with oxaliplatin-cyclophosphamide demonstrated increased CD8+ T-cell infiltration resulting in an increased ratio of CD8+ T cells to regulatory T cells; therefore, sensitizing the tumor microenvironment for immune detection.[9] It has also been shown that expression of PD-L2, a T-cell inhibitor, was downregulated in human tumor cells and dendritic cells after exposure to platinum agents, which led to enhanced antigen-specific proliferation and tumor identification by T cells.[10] Platinum-based chemotherapy also improves tumor cell destruction by granzyme-B–mediated cytotoxic effects of T lymphocytes.[11] Other mechanisms by which platinum agents stimulate the immune system include increasing human leukocyte 1 (HLA1) gene complex expression encoding MHC-I, which is associated with cytotoxic T-cell function.[5] Therefore, based on preclinical studies, there is a strong rationale for combining platinum-based chemotherapy and immunotherapy, and this potential synergistic effect has been demonstrated with improved outcomes in the clinical setting.

CLINICAL DATA COMBINING CHEMOTHERAPY WITH IMMUNOTHERAPY IN NONSQUAMOUS NON–SMALL CELL LUNG CANCER

In patients with metastatic nonsquamous NSCLC, 3 trials, KEYNOTE-189, IMpower150, and IMpower130, have demonstrated improved overall survival (OS) with the addition of an anti-PD-1/PD-L1 antibody to standard chemotherapy (**Table 1**).

Table 1
Major trial data combining chemotherapy with immunotherapy in NSCLC

Name	Description	ORR	mPFS, mo	mOS, mo	HR for OS
Nonsquamous cell					
KeyNote 189[12,20]	Pembrolizumab + chemotherapy vs chemotherapy	48% vs 19%	8.8 vs 4.9	22 .0 vs 10.7 *P*<.00001	0.56
IMPower 150[22]	Atezolizumab + chemotherapy/ bevacizumab vs chemotherapy/ bevacizumab	64% vs 48%	8.3 vs 6.8	19.2 vs 14.7 *P* = .02	0.78
IMPower 130[21]	Atezolizumab + chemotherapy vs chemotherapy	49% vs 32%	7.0 vs 5.5	18.6 vs 13.9 *P* = .033	0.79
Squamous cell					
KeyNote 407[13]	Pembrolizumab + chemotherapy vs chemotherapy	58% vs 38%	6.4 vs 4.8	15.9 vs 11.3 *P*<.001	0.64
IMPower 131[28]	Atezolizumab + chemotherapy vs chemotherapy	59% vs 51%	6.3 vs 5.6	14.0 vs 13.9 *P* = .6931	0.96

Summary of survival data, including mPFS and mOS from the major trials that combined chemotherapy with immunotherapy in both squamous and nonsquamous NSCLC.

Abbreviations: HR, hazard ratio; mOS, median overall survival; mPFS, median progression-free survival; NSCLC, non–small cell lung cancer; ORR, objective response rate; OS, overall survival.

KEYNOTE-189 was a phase III trial of treatment-naïve patients with nonsquamous NSCLC without sensitizing epidermal growth factor receptor (EGFR) or anaplastic large-cell lymphoma kinase (ALK) mutations, who were randomized to receive a platinum and pemetrexed doublet in addition to fixed dose pembrolizumab (200 mg) or placebo.[12,20] This 3-drug combination was administered every 3 weeks for 4 cycles followed by pemetrexed plus pembrolizumab or placebo as maintenance therapy. Outcomes were assessed by an independent central review committee, which demonstrated improved co-primary endpoints, progression-free survival (PFS), and OS. Median PFS was 8.8 months (95% confidence interval [CI] 7.6–9.2) in the pembrolizumab-combination group compared with 4.9 months (95% CI 4.7–5.5) in the placebo-combination group (hazard ratio [HR] for disease progression or death, 0.52; 95% CI 0.43–0.64; *P*<.001). In the updated 18.7-month follow-up analysis, the median OS was 22.0 months in the pembrolizumab arm compared with 10.7 months in the placebo arm (HR 0.56; 95% CI 0.45–0.70; *P*<.00001). Importantly, improvement in OS with immunotherapy and chemotherapy combination was seen across all PD-L1 categories evaluated by tumor proportion score (TPS), including those classified as PD-L1 negative (TPS <1%; HR 0.59; 95% CI 0.39–0.88). The response rate was 47.6% in the pembrolizumab-combination group compared with 18.9% in the placebo-combination group. On disease progression, 50% of the patients randomized to the placebo arm had crossed over to the pembrolizumab arm at the time of analysis. The safety profile was similar with a grade 3 or higher adverse event (AE) occurring in 67.2% of patients in the pembrolizumab arm versus 65.8% of those in the placebo arm. However, more patients discontinued treatment due to an AE in the pembrolizumab-combination group (28% vs 15%). The most common grade 3 or higher adverse events of any cause reported in at least 10% of the patients in the pembrolizumab-combination or the placebo-combination arm were anemia (16.3% vs 15.3%) and neutropenia (15.8% vs 11.9%), which can be attributed to platinum-based combination chemotherapy. As expected, immune-related AEs (irAEs) were more common in the pembrolizumab-combination arm compared with the placebo-combination arm (22.7% vs 11.9%). The most common irAEs of any grade in the pembrolizumab-combination arm compared with the placebo-combination arm were hypothyroidism (6.7% vs 2.5%) and pneumonitis (4.4% vs 2.5%). Grade 3 or higher irAEs occurred in 8.9% of patients in the pembrolizumab-combination arm compared with 4.5% of patients in the placebo-combination arm, the most common of which were pneumonitis (2.7% vs 2.0%) and severe skin reactions (2.0% vs 2.0%). Three patients in the pembrolizumab-combination arm died of pneumonitis. By cross-trial comparison, pembrolizumab combined with chemotherapy did not increase the rate of irAEs compared with pembrolizumab monotherapy given in KEYNOTE-024.[21]

The IMpower130 and the IMpower150 trials both demonstrated OS benefit when atezolizumab was combined with chemotherapy in patients with metastatic nonsquamous NSCLC. Notably, patients with EGFR or ALK mutations who had been treated with 1 or more tyrosine kinase inhibitors (TKIs) were enrolled in both of these studies; however, they were excluded from the primary PFS and OS analysis (intention-to-treat population with wild-type genotype; ITT-WT) in the IMpower 130 study.

IMpower130 was a randomized phase III trial that studied a platinum doublet backbone of carboplatin and nab-paclitaxel with and without atezolizumab (ACnP vs CnP) in patients with metastatic nonsquamous NSCLC.[22] Atezolizumab maintenance was given in the experimental arm and switch maintenance was allowed in the control arm. In the ITT-WT population, a median PFS (7.0 vs 5.5 months; HR 0.64; 95% CI 0.540–.00; *P*<.0001) and OS (18.6 vs 13.9 months; HR 0.79; 95% CI 0.64–0.98; *P* = .033) benefit was demonstrated in the atezolizumab arm. The PFS and OS benefit was seen, consistently, in all PD-L1 subgroups except in patients with liver metastases or EGFR/ALK alterations. The objective response rate (ORR) was 49.2% versus 31.9% in the ACnP versus CnP arms, respectively.

IMpower150 was a phase III trial with 3 treatment arms comparing atezolizumab plus bevacizumab, carboplatin and paclitaxel (ABCP) and atezolizumab plus carboplatin and paclitaxel (ACP) with bevacizumab, carboplatin and paclitaxel (BCP).[23] Four to 6 cycles of carboplatin and paclitaxel were completed, followed by maintenance with atezolizumab, bevacizumab, or both. The median PFS was longer in the ABCP group than in the BCP group in the WT population (8.3 vs 6.8 months; HR 0.62; 95% CI 0.52–0.74; *P*<.001). The PFS benefit was also seen in the entire ITT population, including those with EGFR/ALK genetic alterations, low or negative PD-L1 expression, and those with liver metastases. The median OS in the WT population was also longer in the ABCP group compared with the BCP group (19.2 vs 14.7 months, HR 0.78; 95% CI 0.64–0.96; *P* = .02). Notably, the atezolizumab, carboplatin and paclitaxel (ACP) arm did not show a survival benefit compared with the BCP control arm. The WT population ORR was 63.5% in the ABCP group and 48% in the BCP group; 3.7% of patients in the ABCP group had a complete response compared with 1.2% of the patients in the BCP group.

The magnitude of PFS benefit with immunotherapy was similar in both the IMpower130 trial (7.0 vs 5.5 months with ACnP vs CnP) and IMpower 150 (8.3 vs 6.8 months with ABCP vs BCP).[22,23] The absolute median PFS was longer and ORR was greater with the bevacizumab-containing regimen in the IMpower150 trial. However, the median OS was similar between the IMpower130 (18.6 vs 13.9 months with ACnP vs CnP) and the IMpower 150 (19.2 vs 14.7 months with ABCP vs BCP) trials. The safety profiles of ABCP and ACnP were consistent with previously reported safety risks of the individual medications.

The rate of grade 3 or greater AEs was higher for the 4-drug combination of ABCP than with BCP (58.5% vs 50.0%, respectively) in the IMpower150 trial, but the rate of treatment-related death was similar (2.8% vs 2.3%). As expected, there were more irAEs in the ABCP arm; 77.4% were grade 1 or grade 2 and there were no irAE-associated deaths. The most common irAEs of any grade in the ABCP arm compared with the BCP arm were rash (28.8% vs 13.2%), hepatitis (12.0% vs 7.4%), and hypothyroidism (12.7% vs 3.8%) and grade 3 to 4 irAEs were hepatitis (4.1% vs 0.8%), rash (2.3% vs 0.5%), and pneumonitis (1.5% vs 0.5%).

ROLE OF IMMUNOTHERAPY IN EPIDERMAL GROWTH FACTOR RECEPTOR AND ANAPLASTIC LARGE-CELL LYMPHOMA KINASE MUTATED NON–SMALL CELL LUNG CANCER TUMORS

Earlier randomized trials in patients with EGFR or ALK sensitizing alterations, previously treated with a TKI, indicated that immunotherapy was less effective in the second line compared with patients with WT tumors.[24–26] In fact, in patients with tumors harboring EGFR or ALK alterations, inferior outcomes were observed in those treated with immunotherapy compared with chemotherapy, as first line or after progression on a TKI, regardless of their PD-L1 expression.[27,28] However, in the more recent IMpower 150 trial, PFS benefit was demonstrated in patients with these tumor alterations who had progressive disease after or unacceptable side effects with treatment with at least one approved TKI, who were included in the ITT population, with subsequent treatment including atezolizumab and bevacizumab in addition to a platinum doublet.[23] These data suggest that vascular endothelial growth factor inhibition combined with chemotherapy has immune-modulatory effects, which enhance the efficacy of immunotherapy, resulting in improved survival not typically seen in this subset of patients.

TRIAL DATA COMBINING CHEMOTHERAPY WITH IMMUNOTHERAPY IN SQUAMOUS NON–SMALL CELL LUNG CANCER

In patients with metastatic squamous NSCLC, the KEYNOTE-407 trial demonstrated improved survival in patients treated with the combination of pembrolizumab and a standard platinum doublet (see **Table 1**).[13] This was a phase III trial in treatment-naïve patients randomized to receive carboplatin and the physician's choice of either paclitaxel or nab-paclitaxel in addition to pembrolizumab or placebo for 4 cycles, followed by pembrolizumab or placebo maintenance. There was improvement in the co-primary endpoints, median PFS (6.4 vs 4.8 months, HR 0.56; 95% CI 0.45–0.70; *P*<.001) and median OS (15.9 vs 11.3 months, HR 0.64; 95% CI 0.49–0.85; *P*<.001), in the pembrolizumab arm. The OS benefit was observed regardless of PDL-1 expression. There was also improvement in the ORR with the addition of pembrolizumab compared with placebo (57.9% vs 38.4%, respectively). The incidence of grade 3 or greater AEs was similar in both groups: 69% in the pembrolizumab arm and 68% in the placebo arm. Although there was a higher rate of treatment discontinuation due to AEs in the pembrolizumab arm (23.4%) compared with the placebo arm (11.8%), patients were treated for a longer duration in the pembrolizumab arm (median 6.3 months vs 4.7 months). There were more irAEs in the pembrolizumab arm compared with the placebo arm, as expected, with 28.8% versus 8.6% any grade and 10.8% versus 3.2% grade 3 to 5 irAEs, respectively. The most common irAEs of any grade in the pembrolizumab arm compared with the placebo arm were hypothyroidism (7.9% vs 1.8%), hyperthyroidism (7.2% vs 0.7%), and pneumonitis (6.5% vs 2.1%) and grade 3 to 4 irAEs were pneumonitis (2.5% vs 1.1%), hepatitis (1.8% vs 0%), and infusion reactions (1.4% vs 0.4%). One patient in each arm died of pneumonitis.

Another phase III study, IMpower 131, used the same chemotherapeutic agents combined with atezolizumab but separated into 3 arms: carboplatin with either paclitaxel (ACP) or nab-paclitaxel

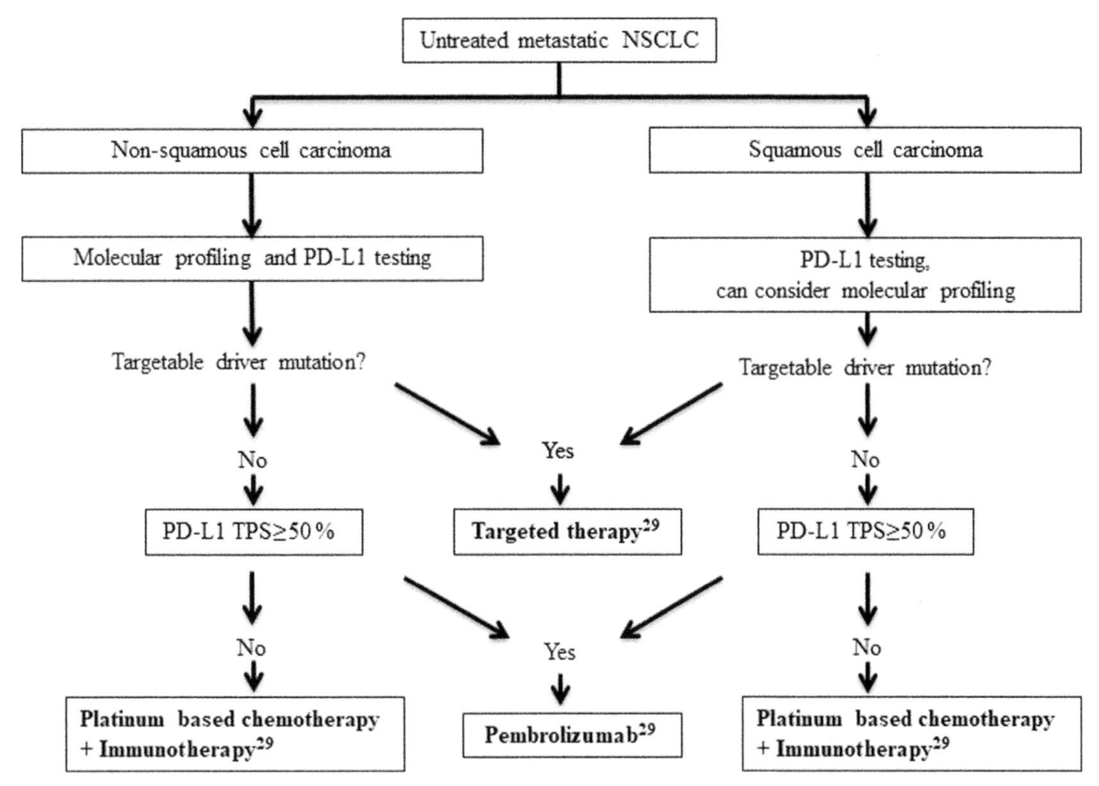

Fig. 1. NSCLC first-line treatment algorithm based on histology and PD-L1 TPS. Histologic subtype must be established with adequate tissue for molecular testing. All nonsquamous cell tumors should have broad molecular profiling. In squamous cell tumors, broad molecular profiling should be considered in never smokers, as they are more likely to have a driver mutation, or in situations in which the histologic diagnosis is less concrete, such as a small biopsy or mixed histology specimen. Patients found to have a driver mutation in EGFR, ALK, ROS1, or BRAF V600 E should receive the respective targeted therapy. All NSCLC tumors must have PD-L1 TPS testing. Those who have a TPS 50% or greater should, generally, be treated with Pembrolizumab monotherapy; however, the addition of platinum-based chemotherapy may be recommended in some situations. If the PD-L1 TPS is less than 50%, at the treating physician's discretion, the patient should be treated with combination platinum-based chemotherapy and immunotherapy.

(ACnP) was compared with carboplatin plus nab-paclitaxel (CnP) alone (see **Table 1**).[29] This study did demonstrate a median PFS benefit with ACnP versus CnP (6.3 vs 5.6 months, respectively; HR 0.71; 95% CI 0.60–0.85; *P*<.0001); however, there was no statistically significant difference in the co-primary endpoint, OS (14.0 vs 13.9 months; HR 0.96; 95% CI 0.78–1.18).

OUTLINE OF ACTIVE TREATMENT PROTOCOLS

Currently, per National Comprehensive Cancer Network guidelines, platinum-based chemotherapy combined with immunotherapy is considered the preferred, category 1, treatment for most cases of advanced or metastatic NSCLC.[30] Patients with metastatic adenocarcinoma, not harboring a driver mutation in EGFR, ALK, ROS1, or BRAF V600 E, and with PDL1 TPS <50%, should receive systemic triplet therapy with carboplatin or cisplatin and pemetrexed combined with pembrolizumab or quadruple therapy with carboplatin, paclitaxel, and bevacizumab combined with atezolizumab, a PD-L1 inhibitor (**Fig. 1**).[12,23] If there is disease response or stable disease per Response Evaluation Criteria in Solid Tumors (RECIST) after 4 cycles of combination therapy, maintenance therapy is continued with pemetrexed and pembrolizumab after triplet therapy or bevacizumab and atezolizumab after quadruple therapy, respectively. First-line, category 1, preferred, systemic therapy options for patients with metastatic squamous cell carcinoma, not harboring the aforementioned driver mutations and with a PD-L1 TPS less than 50%, include pembrolizumab combined with carboplatin and either paclitaxel or nab-paclitaxel (see **Fig. 1**).[13,29] For any patient with metastatic NSCLC whose tumor does not have a driver mutation and has a PD-L1 TPS of ≥50%, the preferred, category 1 treatment is pembrolizumab monotherapy (see **Fig. 1**).[3] There are no currently published trials directly comparing pembrolizumab monotherapy versus combination chemo-immunotherapy in the first-line setting. Therefore, based on clinician discretion, it may be necessary to give combination therapy even in circumstances when the PD-1 TPS is greater than 50%, such as a patient having severely symptomatic disease requiring a time-sensitive response to treatment, or pembrolizumab monotherapy when the PD-L1 TPS is less than 50% if it was felt that the patient would not tolerate chemotherapy.

SUMMARY

During the past decade, there has been significant advancement in the treatment of lung cancer, including the identification of targetable oncogenic driver mutations and more recently with the development of immunotherapeutic agents. It is well established that adaptive immunity plays a major role in the prevention of tumor growth. However, tumor cells exploit mechanisms of self-tolerance, including the PD1/PD-L1 interaction, causing immunosuppression. Antibodies targeting PD-1 and PD-L1 have been developed that enhance the antitumor immune response. Platinum-based chemotherapy has a variety of immune-modulatory effects giving strong rationale for combination treatment with immunotherapy. Chemo-immunotherapy has become the standard of care for most patients with metastatic NSCLC based on durable responses and improved survival. Immunotherapy, specifically durvalumab, has significantly prolonged survival as consolidative therapy in patients with stage III, unresectable NSCLC after concurrent chemoradiotherapy.[31,32] Immunotherapy is now being investigated in earlier-stage disease and preliminary data suggest impressive responses to chemo-immunotherapy in the neoadjuvant setting for resectable stage IB-IIIA NSCLC.[33] The future of NSCLC therapy will be reliant on the durable tumor control provided with immunotherapy, as well as a combinatorial agent to enhance antitumor immunity and cancer cell death.

DISCLOSURE

J. Judd has nothing to disclose. H. Borghaei has research support from Millennium, Merck/Celgene, and BMS/Lilly; Advisory Board role/Consultant for BMS, Lilly, Genentech, Celgene, Pfizer, Merck, EMD-Serono, Boehringer Ingelheim, Astra Zeneca, Novartis, Genmab, Regeneron, BioNTech, Cantargia AB, Amgen, AbbVie, Axiom, PharmaMar, Takeda, Huya Bio; and Data and Safety Monitoring Board role with University of Pennsylvania CAR T Program and Takeda.

REFERENCES

1. Jemal A, Bray F, Center MM, et al. Global cancer statistics. CA Cancer J Clin 2011;61(2):69–90.
2. Siegel RL, Miller KD, Jemal A. Cancer statistics, 2018. CA Cancer J Clin 2018;68(1):7–30.
3. Reck M, Rodríguez-Abreu D, Robinson AG, et al. Pembrolizumab versus chemotherapy for PD-L1-positive non-small-cell lung cancer. N Engl J Med 2016;375(19):1823–33.
4. Davies J, Patel M, Gridelli C, et al. Real-world treatment patterns for patients receiving second-line and third-line treatment for advanced non-small cell lung

cancer: a systematic review of recently published studies. PLoS One 2017;12(4):e0175679.
5. Liu WM, Fowler DW, Smith P, et al. Pre-treatment with chemotherapy can enhance the antigenicity and immunogenicity of tumours by promoting adaptive immune responses. Br J Cancer 2010;102(1):115–23.
6. Kroemer G, Galluzzi L, Kepp O, et al. Immunogenic cell death in cancer therapy. Annu Rev Immunol 2013;31:51–72.
7. Tseng CW, Hung CF, Alvarez RD, et al. Pretreatment with cisplatin enhances E7-specific CD8+ T-Cell-mediated antitumor immunity induced by DNA vaccination. Clin Cancer Res 2008;14(10):3185–92.
8. Suzuki E, Kapoor V, Jassar AS, et al. Gemcitabine selectively eliminates splenic Gr-1+/CD11b+ myeloid suppressor cells in tumor-bearing animals and enhances antitumor immune activity. Clin Cancer Res 2005;11(18):6713–21.
9. Pfirschke C, Engblom C, Rickelt S, et al. Immunogenic chemotherapy sensitizes tumors to checkpoint blockade therapy. Immunity 2016;44(2):343–54.
10. Lesterhuis WJ, Punt CJ, Hato SV, et al. Platinum-based drugs disrupt STAT6-mediated suppression of immune responses against cancer in humans and mice. J Clin Invest 2011;121(8):3100–8.
11. Ramakrishnan R, Assudani D, Nagaraj S, et al. Chemotherapy enhances tumor cell susceptibility to CTL-mediated killing during cancer immunotherapy in mice. J Clin Invest 2010;120(4):1111–24.
12. Gandhi L, Rodríguez-Abreu D, Gadgeel S, et al. Pembrolizumab plus chemotherapy in metastatic non-small-cell lung cancer. N Engl J Med 2018;378(22):2078–92.
13. Paz-Ares L, Luft A, Vicente D, et al. Pembrolizumab plus chemotherapy for squamous non-small-cell lung cancer. N Engl J Med 2018;379(21):2040–51.
14. Dalgleish AG, O'Byrne K. Inflammation and cancer: the role of the immune response and angiogenesis. Cancer Treat Res 2006;130:1–38.
15. Chen DS, Mellman I. Oncology meets immunology: the cancer-immunity cycle. Immunity 2013;39(1):1–10.
16. Hanahan D, Weinberg RA. The hallmarks of cancer. Cell 2000;100(1):57–70.
17. Pardoll DM. The blockade of immune checkpoints in cancer immunotherapy. Nat Rev Cancer 2012;12(4):252–64.
18. Chen DS, Irving BA, Hodi FS. Molecular pathways: next-generation immunotherapy–inhibiting programmed death-ligand 1 and programmed death-1. Clin Cancer Res 2012;18(24):6580–7.
19. Butte MJ, Keir ME, Phamduy TB, et al. Programmed death-1 ligand 1 interacts specifically with the B7-1 costimulatory molecule to inhibit T cell responses. Immunity 2007;27(1):111–22.
20. Gadgeel SM, Garassino MC, Esteban E, et al. KEYNOTE-189: updated OS and progression after the next line of therapy (PFS2) with pembrolizumab (pembro) plus chemo with pemetrexed and platinum vs placebo plus chemo for metastatic nonsquamous NSCLC. J Clin Oncol 2019;37(15_suppl):9013.
21. Reck M, Rodríguez-Abreu D, Robinson AG, et al. Updated analysis of KEYNOTE-024: pembrolizumab versus platinum-based chemotherapy for advanced non-small-cell lung cancer with PD-L1 tumor proportion score of 50% or greater. J Clin Oncol 2019;37(7):537–46.
22. Cappuzzo F, McCleod M, Hussein M, et al. IMpower130: progression-free survival (PFS) and safety analysis from a randomised phase III study of carboplatin + nab-paclitaxel (CnP) with or without atezolizumab (atezo) as first-line (1L) therapy in advanced non-squamous NSCLC. Ann Oncol 2018;29(suppl_8) [Abstract nr LBA53].
23. Socinski MA, Jotte RM, Cappuzzo F, et al. Atezolizumab for first-line treatment of metastatic nonsquamous NSCLC. N Engl J Med 2018;378(24):2288–301.
24. Herbst RS, Baas P, Kim DW, et al. Pembrolizumab versus docetaxel for previously treated, PD-L1-positive, advanced non-small-cell lung cancer (KEYNOTE-010): a randomised controlled trial. Lancet 2016;387(10027):1540–50.
25. Borghaei H, Paz-Ares L, Horn L, et al. Nivolumab versus docetaxel in advanced nonsquamous non-small-cell lung cancer. N Engl J Med 2015;373(17):1627–39.
26. Fehrenbacher L, Spira A, Ballinger M, et al. Atezolizumab versus docetaxel for patients with previously treated non-small-cell lung cancer (POPLAR): a multicentre, open-label, phase 2 randomised controlled trial. Lancet 2016;387(10030):1837–46.
27. Peters S, Gettinger S, Johnson ML, et al. Phase II trial of atezolizumab as first-line or subsequent therapy for patients with programmed death-ligand 1-selected advanced non-small-cell lung cancer (BIRCH). J Clin Oncol 2017;35(24):2781–9.
28. Haratani K, Hayashi H, Tanaka T, et al. Tumor immune microenvironment and nivolumab efficacy in EGFR mutation-positive non-small-cell lung cancer based on T790M status after disease progression during EGFR-TKI treatment. Ann Oncol 2017;28(7):1532–9.
29. Jotte RM. IMpower131: primary PFS and safety analysis of a randomized phase III study of atezolizumab þ carboplatin + paclitaxel or nab-paclitaxel vs carboplatin + nab-paclitaxel as 1L therapy in advanced squamous NSCLC. J Clin Oncol 2018;36(suppl) [abstract LBA9000].
30. National Comprehensive Cancer Network. Non-small cell lung cancer (version 5.2019). 2019. Available at: https://www.nccn.org/professionals/physician_gls/pdf/nscl.pdf. Accessed July 15, 2019.
31. Antonia SJ, Villegas A, Daniel D, et al. Durvalumab after chemoradiotherapy in stage III

non-small-cell lung cancer. N Engl J Med 2017; 377(20):1919–29.
32. Antonia SJ, Villegas A, Daniel D, et al. Overall survival with durvalumab after chemoradiotherapy in stage III NSCLC. N Engl J Med 2018;379(24): 2342–50.
33. Provencio M, Nadal E, Insa A, et al. Neoadjuvant chemo-immunotherapy for the treatment of stage IIIA resectable non-small-cell lung cancer (NSCLC): a phase II multicenter exploratory study—Final data of patients who underwent surgical assessment. J Clin Oncol 2019;37(15_suppl):8509.

Biomarkers for Immunotherapy

Jean G. Bustamante-Alvarez, MD, MS, Dwight H. Owen, MD, MS*

KEYWORDS

• Biomarkers • Immunotherapy • Checkpoint inhibitor • PD-L1 • Non–small cell lung cancer (NSCLC)

KEY POINTS

- Programmed death-ligand 1 (PD-L1) is currently the only biomarker approved for use by the US Food and Drug Administration (FDA) to guide treatment decisions specifically in non–small cell lung cancer (NSCLC), and it predicts response to anti–programmed cell death protein 1 (PD-1) and anti–PD-L1 blockade in NSCLC without driver mutations such as *EGFR* or *ALK* mutations.
- High tumor mutation burden suggests an increased neoantigen load and has been associated with increased likelihood for clinical benefit from ICI therapy.
- Microsatellite instability is an FDA-approved biomarker for ICI therapy across solid tumors, but it is uncommon in NSCLC.
- Although no 1 mutation seems to drive response or resistance to treatment, subsets of patients with mutations in serine/threonine kinase 11 (*STK11*) and *EGFR* genes seem to be less likely to benefit from ICI therapy.
- Resistance to immune checkpoint inhibitors can be primary and mediated by mutations such as *STK11/LKB1* mutations, or acquired in several pathways, including genomic immunoediting resulting in the depletion of potentially immunogenic neoantigens; truncation of JAK-1/JAK2 proteins altering the signaling pathway; and mutations that render beta2-microglobulin (invariant chain of the major histocompatibility complex I) defective, altering antigen presentation.

INTRODUCTION

Biomarkers in the immunotherapy era are important to select the groups of patients who are likely to benefit from anti–programmed cell death protein 1 (PD-1) and anti–programmed death-ligand 1 (PD-L1) immune checkpoint inhibitors (ICIs). To date, the only US Food and Drug Administration (FDA)–approved biomarkers to decide which frontline treatment patients with advanced non–small cell lung cancer (NSCLC) receive are PD-L1 tumor proportion score (TPS) in cancer cells and microsatellite instability. Other promising markers being investigated include tumor mutation burden (TMB), tumor infiltrating lymphocytes (TILs), and density of CD8+ cells in the tumor microenvironment. The genomic landscape of the tumor affects immunogenicity and the response to ICIs. This article discusses how these factors affect immune response as well as recent advances and future directions that are defining better strategies to predict outcomes with ICIs in patients with advanced NSCLC.

TUMOR EXPRESSION OF PROGRAMMED DEATH-LIGAND 1 BY IMMUNOHISTOCHEMISTRY

PD-L1 is a transmembrane protein encoded by the *PD-L1* gene found in chromosome 9 in humans. Its expression can be constitutive at low levels on resting lymphocytes, antigen-presenting cells (APCs), and other tissues contributing to homeostasis in proinflammatory states.[1] PD-1 is an

Division of Medical Oncology, Department of Internal Medicine, Ohio State University Wexner Medical Center, 320 West 10th Avenue, A450B Starling Loving Hall, Columbus, OH 43210, USA
* Corresponding author.
E-mail address: Dwight.owen@osumc.edu

Thorac Surg Clin 30 (2020) 207–214
https://doi.org/10.1016/j.thorsurg.2020.01.010

inhibitory molecule present on B cells, activated T cells, and natural killer cells that binds to PD-L1 (also known as B7-H1 or CD271) and PD-L2 (also known as B7-DC or CD273) expressed in tumor cells and APCs.[2] The interaction of PD-1 with its ligand PD-L1 inhibits the proliferation, survival, and effector activity of cytotoxic T lymphocytes, induces apoptosis of tumor-infiltrating lymphocytes (TILs), and increases the microenvironment recruitment of immunosuppressive regulatory T cells.[3] In advanced NSCLC, approximately 40% to 58% of the patient are PD-L1 negative, 28% to 31% are PD-L1 low (≥1% to ≤49%), and 10% to 32% have high PD-L1 expression (≥50%).[4,5] Immune checkpoint blockade of the PD-1/PD-L1 axis has revolutionized the treatment of NSCLC, becoming a standard-of-care treatment option for patients in the frontline setting alone or in combination with chemotherapy.[6]

PD-L1 is measured by immunohistochemistry (IHC), and 5 different anti–PD-L1 immunoglobulin G1 antibodies have been used for testing across clinical trials: 22C3, 28-8, SP142, SP263, and 73-10. The percentage of expression is most commonly measured using the TPS, which is estimated by the manual quantification of viable tumor cells with cell membrane staining (partial or complete) of greater than or equal to 1+ intensity.[7]

Multiple clinical trials have tested PD-1 and PD-L1 inhibitors, showing the value of PD-L1 as a predictive biomarker. KEYNOTE-010 was a randomized, open-label, phase 2/3 clinical trial that compared pembrolizumab at 2 different doses (2 or 10 mg/kg every 3 weeks) with docetaxel in previously treated patients with advanced NSCLC with at least 1% PD-L1 TPS. The primary end points were overall survival (OS) and progression-free survival (PFS). Pembrolizumab-treated patients had a significantly longer OS compared with patients treated with docetaxel in the overall study population (OS 10.4 months with pembrolizumab 2 mg/kg, hazard ratio [HR] 0.71, *P* = .008; 12.7 months with pembrolizumab 10 mg/kg, HR 0.61, *P*<.0001; and 8.5 months with docetaxel). At 1 year, a higher percentage of patients treated with pembrolizumab were alive compared with those treated with docetaxel (OS 52.3% for pembrolizumab 10 mg/kg versus 43.2% for pembrolizumab 2 mg/kg versus 34.6% for docetaxel). Higher PD-L1 TPS was predictive of longer survival in a subgroup analysis (PD-L1 TPS ≥50% HR for death 0.53 compared with 0.76 for TPS 1%–49%). The median OS for patients with TPS PD-L1 greater than or equal to 50% was 14.9 months versus 8.2 months (HR, 0.54; 95% confidence interval [CI], 0.38–0·77; *P* = .0002) for the pembrolizumab 2 mg/kg group and docetaxel groups respectively, and 17.3 months versus 8.2 months (HR, 0.50; 95% CI, 0.36–0.70; *P*<.0001) for the pembrolizumab 10 mg/kg group and docetaxel group.[8]

KEYNOTE-024 was a phase 3 trial that evaluated pembrolizumab monotherapy compared with standard-of-care platinum-based doublet chemotherapy in the first-line setting for epidermal growth factor receptor (EGFR)–negative and anaplastic lymphoma kinase (ALK)–negative advanced NSCLC with PD-L1 TPS greater than or equal to 50%. The primary objective of this study was PFS. This trial showed a clear benefit for those patients treated with immunotherapy in terms of median PFS, OS, and response rates. Median duration of response was not reached in the pembrolizumab arm.[5,9,10] Long-term follow-up results were recently published for KEYNOTE-024, and the median OS reported for patients treated with first-line pembrolizumab was 30.0 months (95% CI, 18.3 months; not reached) with pembrolizumab and 14.2 months (95% CI, 9.8–19.0 months) with chemotherapy.[9] This trial ultimately led to the approval of pembrolizumab monotherapy for patients with metastatic NSCLC with high expression of PD-L1 (≥50%) without actionable mutations (**Table 1**).

KEYNOTE-042 was a phase 3 trial that led to the approval of pembrolizumab for PD-L1–positive advanced NSCLC with any level of PD-L1 expression. KEYNOTE-042 was a randomized, open-label, international, multicenter, double-blinded clinical trial of pembrolizumab monotherapy compared with standard-of-care chemotherapy in patients with untreated metastatic NSCLC with PD-L1–positive tumors (ie, TPS ≥ 1%). The intention-to-treat population showed significantly longer OS in patients who received pembrolizumab compared with chemotherapy in the first ine in all PD-L1 TPS groups (PD-L1 ≥ 50%, HR 0.69, 95% CI 0.56–0.85, *P* = .0003; PD-L1 ≥ 20%, HR 0.77, 95% CI, 0.64–0.92, *P* = .0020; and PD-L1 ≥ 1%, HR 0.81, 95% CI 0.71–0.93, *P* = .0018). Median survival values were 20.0 months (95% CI 15.4–24.9) for pembrolizumab versus 12.2 months (95% CI 10·4–14·2) for chemotherapy in the greater than or equal to 50% population, 17.7 months (95% CI 15.3–22.1) versus 13.0 months (95% CI 11.6–15.3) in the ≥20% population, and 16.7 months (95% CI 13.9–19.7) versus 12.1 months (95% CI 11.3–13.3) in the greater than or equal to 1% population, respectively.[10]

Across most immunotherapy clinical trials with ICI in *EGFR* mutation–negative and *ALK* mutation–negative advanced NSCLC, high levels of PD-L1 expression have been correlated with better PFS, OS, and response rates compared

Table 1
Approved and investigational biomarkers for immune checkpoint inhibitor therapy in non–small cell lung cancer

FDA-Approved Biomarkers	Intervention	Outcomes	Clinical Trial and Evidence
PD-L1 ≥ 50%	Pembrolizumab first line vs chemotherapy	Longer PFS and OS with pembrolizumab	KEYNOTE-024[9] KEYNOTE-407[41]
PD-L1 ≥ 1%	Pembrolizumab first line	Longer OS	KEYNOTE-042[10]
MSI-H	Pembrolizumab any histology	Improved response rates, PFS and OS compared with MSS	Le et al,[24] 2015
Investigational Biomarkers	**Intervention**	**Outcomes**	**Clinical Trial and Evidence**
TMB high (per foundation)	Nivolumab/ ipilimumab	Improved response rates and PFS	CheckMate-227[20] and CheckMate-026[18]
STK11/LKB1 mutated	Anti–PD-1 or anti–PD-L1 or anti–PD-L1 plus anti–CTLA-4	Shorter PFS	SU2C and CheckMate-057[30]
HLA class I allele C03:04	ICI	Shorter PFS	Negrao et al,[37] 2019
Acquired beta2-microglobulin loss	Anti–PD-L1 plus anti-CTLA antibodies	Resistance to ICIs	Gettinger et al,[36] 2017

Abbreviations: CTLA-4, cytotoxic T lymphocyte–associated protein 4; HLA, human leukocyte antigen; MSS, microsatellite stable; MSI-H, microsatellite instability high.

with chemotherapy in the first-line setting.[9–11] Of note, both nivolumab (anti–PD-1 monoclonal antibody) and atezolizumab (anti–PD-L1 monoclonal antibody) are approved in the second-line setting for patients with metastatic NSCLC who have progressed on platinum-doublet chemotherapy regardless of PD-L1 expression.[12–15]

TUMOR MUTATIONAL BURDEN

TMB is the composite of somatic nonsynonymous mutations (insertions, deletions, and somatic protein-coding base substitutions) per coding area of a tumor genome.[16] Increased mutational load can result from exposure to ultraviolet rays, smoking, and other environmental and nutritional compounds that lead to inflammation.[17] Mutational load can also increase as a result of defects in the proofreading domains of DNA polymerases.[17] High TMB has been hypothesized to enhance immunogenicity by increasing the neoantigens expressed by the cancer cells that are recognized by T cells as foreign, triggering a more robust immune response in the presence of ICIs (see **Table 1**).[16,18]

TMB has been measured with different methods, including whole-exome sequencing (WES) and targeted next-generation sequencing (NGS) panels. Rizvi and colleagues[19] used WES to determine TMB in patients with NSCLC and reported an association between higher somatic nonsynonymous mutation burden and clinical efficacy of pembrolizumab in 2 different cohorts of patients. The discovery cohort was composed of 16 patients and had a median number of nonsynonymous mutations for patients with durable clinical benefit lasting longer than 6 months of 302 versus 148 for the group with no durable benefit ($P = .02$). More patients with high nonsynonymous burden, defined as greater than the median burden of the cohort (209), experienced durable clinical benefit compared with those with low mutation burden (73% vs 13% respectively, $P = .04$). In patients with high nonsynonymous mutation burden, improved response rates and PFS were also observed (OR of response [ORR] 63% vs 0%, $P = .03$; median PFS 14.5 vs 3.7 months, $P = .01$; HR 0.19, 95% CI 0.05–0.70). An independent set of 18 NSCLC samples from patients treated with pembrolizumab composed the validation cohort. The median nonsynonymous mutation burden was 244 in tumors from patients with durable clinical benefit compared with 125 in those with nondurable clinical benefit (P = .04). PFS was significantly longer in patients with a nonsynonymous mutation burden greater than 200, the median of the validation cohort (median PFS not reached vs 3.4 months, P = .006; HR 0.15, 95% CI 0.04–0.59).[19]

Subsequently, in an exploratory analysis of TMB conducted as part of the CheckMate-026 study, TMB was calculated with WES on tumor and matched whole-blood DNA in 312 patients. Patients were grouped in thirds according to TMB. A TMB of 0 to less than 100 mutations was considered low burden, 100 to 242 mutations medium burden, and 243 or more mutations high burden. Patients with a high TMB treated with nivolumab had higher response rates (47% vs 28%) and longer PFS (median, 9.7 vs 5.8 months; HR for disease progression or death, 0.62; 95% CI, 0.38–1.00) compared with patients treated with chemotherapy.[18]

CheckMate-227 was a phase 3 open-label multiarm clinical trial that compared nivolumab, nivolumab plus ipilimumab (anti–cytotoxic T lymphocyte–associated protein 4 [CTLA-4] antibody), and nivolumab plus platinum-doublet chemotherapy with platinum-doublet chemotherapy in patients with stage IV NSCLC. TMB was calculated with a targeted NGS panel after application of various filters and was ultimately divided by the region counted (0.8 Mb) to yield mutations per megabase. A prespecified cutoff for TMB of 10 mutations per megabase was selected for preplanned analysis of PFS with nivolumab plus ipilimumab versus chemotherapy in a patient population selected by tumor mutational burden. Patients who received treatment with combined PD-1 and CTLA-4 had higher response rates (45.3% vs 26.9%) than those treated with chemotherapy. At 1 year, the PFS rate was 42.6% with nivolumab plus ipilimumab versus 13.2% with chemotherapy. Median PFS was 7.2 months (95% CI, 5.5–13.2) versus 5.5 months (95% CI, 4.4–5.8; HR for disease progression or death, 0.58; 97.5% CI, 0.41–0.81; P<.001).[20]

Samstein and colleagues[21] found that TMB predicted survival after immunotherapy across multiple cancer types when calculated with the MSK-IMPACT [Memorial Sloan Kettering- Integrated Mutation Profiling of Actionable Cancer Targets] assay, which is a targeted NGS-based method. This study included 350 patients with NSCLC who had received ICIs. The cutoff defining the top 30% of normalized mutational burden from MSK-IMPACT for NSCLC was 10.8 mutations per megabase. Patients within this group had better OS (HR, 0.75; P<.032). In summary, TMB is an emerging biomarker that has been shown to predict response to ICI treatment in several clinical trials. Higher mutational load in tumors likely increases the probability that resulting neoantigens are immunogenic and trigger a prominent antitumoral response, but harmonization of the methods to measure TMB is necessary to better apply this biomarker in clinical practice and select better for patients who will benefit from ICIs.

MICROSATELLITE INSTABILITY AND MISMATCH REPAIR–DEFICIENT CANCERS

The DNA mismatch repair (MMR) process, when defective, leads to a hypermutated genomic status called microsatellite instability high (MSI-H). MMR proteins include mutL homolog 1 (MLH1), MutS homolog 2 (MSH2), mutS homolog 6 (MSH6) and PMS1 Homolog 2 (PMS2), and inactivation of any of the encoding genes occurs as a result of somatic mutations in 80% of the cases and 20% are secondary to germline mutations (Lynch syndrome) that are followed by a second inactivating somatic change in the remaining wild-type allele.[17,22] MMR-deficient colorectal cancers have up to 100 times more somatic mutations than MMR-proficient colorectal adenocarcinomas, and MMR-deficient cancers have prominent lymphocyte infiltrates that also correlate with immune response.[22] MSI-H tumors show upregulation of checkpoints within the tumor microenvironment, including PD-1, PD-L1, lymphocyte activation gene 3 (LAG3), and indolamine 2,3-dioxygenase (IDO). These checkpoints counterbalance the activity of CD8+ cytotoxic T lymphocytes that infiltrate the tumor microenvironment found in MMR-deficient malignancies.[23] A phase 2 study compared outcomes between pembrolizumab-treated patients with MMR-deficient solid tumors and patients treated with pembrolizumab who had MMR-proficient solid tumors. WES showed approximately 1782 somatic mutations per tumor in patients with MMR-deficient cancer and an average of 73 mutations per tumor in patients with MMR-proficient cancer (P = .007). Observed ORR was 39.6% among 149 patients with 15 different tumor types (95% CI, 31.7, 47.9), of which 7% had a complete response. Four out of 10 patients with MMR-deficient colorectal cancer responded to pembrolizumab (see **Table 1**).[24] Based on this study, pembrolizumab was FDA approved for the treatment of adult and pediatric patients with unresectable or metastatic, microsatellite MSI-H, or MMR-deficient solid tumors who have no satisfactory alternative treatment options after progression to prior treatments.[22]

TUMOR LYMPHOCYTE INFILTRATION

Tumor lymphocyte infiltration has been correlated with a better survival in surgical patients when the CD4+/CD8+ T-cell ratio was greater. In the LACE-Bio (Lung Adjuvant Cisplatin Evaluation Biomarker) study, intense versus nonintense tumor lymphocyte infiltration was studied, the primary end point being the OS, and secondary end point the disease-free survival (DFS) and specific DFS. The patients on this trial had localized NSCLC. Intense lymphocyte infiltration was defined as more than 50% stromal lymphocytes in the tumor bulk compared with epithelial tumor cells. This study showed tumor lymphocyte infiltration as an independent prognostic factor, predicting that those patients who had intense tumor lymphocyte infiltration had longer OS. Adjusted HRs for OS, DFS, and specific DFS were 0.56, 0.59, and 0.56 respectively for patients with intense lymphocyte infiltration.[25]

MULTIOMICS PREDICTION MODEL FOR IMMUNE CHECKPOINT INHIBITOR RESPONSE

Given the complexity of host-tumor immune interactions, it is likely that 1 biomarker alone will not be sufficient to guide treatment selection. Instead, it may be that a combination of biomarkers is needed. In 1 study, Lee and Ruppin[26] found that a trivariate model composed of TMB, estimated CD8+ T-cell abundance (eCD8T), and fraction of high PD-1 messenger RNA expression samples (fPD1) enhanced the prediction of the response to anti–PD-1/PD-l1 therapy across different tumor types. In this study, 21 cancer types were studied. TMB and ORR had a high and significant correlation (Spearman $R = 0.68$; $P<6.2 \times 10^{-4}$). eCD8T was the strongest positive correlate of ORR ($R = 0.72$; $P<2.3 \times 10^{-4}$). Most cancer types with higher response rates than that predicted by the TMB regression model had higher eCD8T levels, and those showing lower responses than TMB-based predicted model had lower eCD8T levels. When combining the TMB and eCD8T model, the response prediction was markedly enhanced ($R = 0.85$; $P<1.1 \times 10^{-6}$) showing an improved and significant log-likelihood model compared with univariate models ($P<.001$). When fPD1 was added to the bivariate mutational burden–eCD8T model, the resulting trivariate regression model had significantly improved accuracy ($R = 0.90$; $P < 4.1 \times 10^{-8}$; log-likelihood ratio test $P < .02$). Those cancer subtypes with a higher response than that predicted by the bivariate prediction model had higher fPD1 levels, and those with lower responses had lower fPD1 levels.

MUTATIONAL STATUS

Patients with different oncogenes seem to have varying responses to ICI therapy, which may be caused by a variety of factors. For instance, *EGFR*-mutated tumors have been reported to have an inverse relationship with PD-L1 expression, low mutation burden, lack of T-cell infiltration, and decreased proportion of PD-L1+/CD8+ TILs ($P = .034$).[27] In a prospective phase 2 trial of pembrolizumab in patients with *EGFR*-mutated NSCLC, no objective responses were observed in patients with sensitizing EGFR mutations.[28]

A multicenter international retrospective study (IMMUNOTARGET) analyzed 551 patients from 24 centers from 10 countries with driver mutations including *KRAS*, *EGFR*-activating mutations, *ALK* rearrangement, *ROS1* rearrangement, *BRAF* (exon 15 mutation), *RET* rearrangement, *MET* amplification or exon 14 mutation, and *HER2* (exon 20)-activating mutation. Ninety-four percent of the patients received an anti–PD-1 antibody and 6% an anti–PD-L1 antibody. Only 5% of patients received ICI as first line and 40% as second line; the rest received ICI as third line and beyond. The percentage of PD-L1 expression according to driver mutation was 0 in *HER2* (n = 13), 3.5 in *EGFR* (n = 38), 7.5 in *ALK* (n = 10), 12.5 in *KRAS* (n = 80), 26 in *RET* (n = 6), 30 in *MET* (n = 15), 50 in *BRAF* (n = 9), and 90 in *ROS1* (n = 5). The ORR by driver alteration was *KRAS* 26%, *BRAF* 24%, *ROS1* 17%, *MET* 16%, *EGFR* 12%, *HER2* 7%, *RET* 6%, and *ALK* 0%. For *KRAS*-mutant patients, there was no difference in terms of PFS between *KRAS* mutation subtype and smoking status. However, PD-L1 positivity was significantly ($P = .01$) correlated with a longer PFS (median PFS, 7.2 vs 3.9 months). Patients with *BRAF* (4.1 vs 1.9 months, $P = .03$)-mutated and *HER2* (3.4 months vs 2.0 months, $P = .04$)-mutated tumors who were also smokers had longer PFS compared with never smokers. Rearranged tumors (*ALK*, *ROS1*, and *RET*) with PD-L1 positivity did not have any reported response to ICIs, and median PFS in never smokers (2.6 months) was slightly increased compared with smokers (1.8 months, $P = .03$).[29]

STK11/LKB1

Serine/threonine-protein kinase/liver kinase B1 (*STK11/LKB1*) is a tumor suppressor inactivated in approximately one-third of *KRAS*-mutated lung adenocarcinomas and represents an important primary resistance mechanism to ICIs. The *STK11/LKB1* gene encodes for a serine threonine kinase that, when inactivated by mutational or nonmutational mechanisms, can affect the tumor immune microenvironment, leading to reduced infiltrating cytotoxic CD8+ T lymphocytes in both human tumors and genetically engineered murine models.[30] Mouse models genetically ablated for this gene also showed increased accumulation in the expression of T-cell exhaustion markers, and secretion of interleukin-6 by tumor cells, which leads to recruitment of myeloid cells and neutrophils with suppressive T-cell capabilities. PD-L1 expression was negatively affected by *LKB1* loss in lung cancer cells in mouse and human tumors and cell lines. Depletion of neutrophils and neutralization of interleukin-6 in mouse models with *STK11/LKB1* loss increased T-cell function and number.[31] STK11/LKB1 is also an upstream activator of the adenosine monophosphate-activated protein kinase (AMPK) signaling pathway, which, if inactive, cannot inhibit the mammalian target of rapamycin (mTOR) pathway or induce mitochondrial autophagy. The unrestrained mTOR pathway ultimately results in a growth advantage to cancer cells. *LKB1* loss promotes the suppression of stimulator interferon genes (STINGs) as a result of enhanced DNMT1 and EZH2 expression and activity. STINGs also promote downstream activation of the effector TBK1-IRF3 pathway, producing type I interferons and other cytotoxic mechanisms such as STAT-2 effector programs. Reinduction of LKB1 and STING restored PD-L1 cancer cell surface levels and led to increased T-cell chemotaxis by induction of *CXCL10* expression.[32]

Retrospective clinical studies from 2 different cohorts of patients (SU2C and CheckMate-057) have shown that STK11/LKB1 alteration renders lung adenocarcinomas less responsive to PD-1 blockade with evident lower ORR, PFS ($P<.001$), and OS ($P = .0015$) compared with lung adenocarcinomas with *KRAS* mutations but wild-type *STK11/LKB1*.[30]

SMOKING HISTORY

In a study by Borghei and colleagues,[12] patients treated with nivolumab who were current or former smokers had an OS benefit compared with nonsmokers with advanced nonsquamous NSCLC. Two studies correlated smoking history with increased TPS for PD-L1.[33–35] A study by Rizvi and colleagues[19] analyzed the ORR in patients treated with immunotherapy according to the presence of a smoking gene signature. The group harboring the smoking gene signature had higher ORR compared with the group of patients without it (56% vs 17%, $P = .03$).[19] In addition, an analysis of KEYNOTE-024 indicated survival gains of smoking cessation during immunotherapy.[5]

HUMAN LEUKOCYTE ANTIGEN CLASS I

Human leukocyte antigen (HLA) class I has a role in antitumor immune response and a broader repertoire of these molecules should translate into increased odds of immunogenic antigen presentation and probability of response to ICIs. Major histocompatibility complex I (MHC-I) corresponds in humans to HLA-A, HLA-B, and HLA-C. Decreased expression of beta2-microglobulin, which is a component of MHC-I, has been described as an acquired resistance mechanism to ICIs.[36] However, a recent study conducted at MD Anderson Cancer Center that evaluated 3 independent cohorts of patients with advanced NSCLC treated with PD-1/PD-L1 therapies showed no difference in outcomes based on HLA status. The study investigators evaluated PD-L1 expression, TMB, HLA genotyping, mutational status, and the presence of *STK11* mutations other than synonymous alterations and correlated these biomarkers with patient outcomes. HLA typing was performed and 2 groups were defined: HLA heterozygous if the patients were heterozygous for all HLA class I loci and homozygous if homozygous for at least 1 HLA class I locus. HLA-A and HLA-B were grouped into supertypes. There was no statistically significant difference in PFS between HLA heterozygous and homozygous patients.[37]

FUTURE DIRECTIONS

Several biomarkers have been evaluated to determine the correlation with anti–PD-1 therapies and long-term outcome. TMB, PD-L1, and CD8 have each been associated with benefit from PD-1 blockade. Pretreatment PD-L1 expression has been correlated with T-lymphocyte infiltration and OS. Analysis of a composite of 3 biomarkers seems to have the potential to determine the long-term outcomes for those patients receiving immunotherapy.[38] Soluble PD-L1 and TMB in blood are also being evaluated as biomarkers for selection of candidates who will benefit from immunotherapy.[39,40] In addition, biomarkers for the emergence of secondary resistance need to be identified to identify patients who need either additional or a change in therapy to sustain a clinical benefit.

DISCLOSURE

DHO is a supported by the Paul Calabresi Career Development Award for Clinical Oncology (K12CA133250).

REFERENCES

1. Kythreotou A, Siddique A, Mauri FA, et al. Pd-L1. J Clin Pathol 2018;71(3):189–94.
2. Bustamante Alvarez JG, Gonzalez-Cao M, Karachaliou N, et al. Advances in immunotherapy for treatment of lung cancer. Cancer Biol Med 2015;12(3):209–22.
3. Karwacz K, Bricogne C, MacDonald D, et al. PD-L1 co-stimulation contributes to ligand-induced T cell receptor down-modulation on CD8+ T cells. EMBO Mol Med 2011;3(10):581–92.
4. Velcheti V, Patwardhan PD, Liu FX, et al. Real-world PD-L1 testing and distribution of PD-L1 tumor expression by immunohistochemistry assay type among patients with metastatic non-small cell lung cancer in the United States. PLoS One 2018; 13(11):e0206370.
5. Reck M, Rodriguez-Abreu D, Robinson AG, et al. Pembrolizumab versus chemotherapy for PD-L1-positive non-small-cell lung cancer. N Engl J Med 2016;375(19):1823–33.
6. Ettinger DS, Aisner DL, Wood DE, et al. NCCN guidelines insights: non-small cell lung cancer, version 5.2018. J Natl Compr Canc Netw 2018; 16(7):807–21.
7. Teixido C, Vilarino N, Reyes R, et al. PD-L1 expression testing in non-small cell lung cancer. Ther Adv Med Oncol 2018;10. 1758835918763493.
8. Herbst RS, Baas P, Kim DW, et al. Pembrolizumab versus docetaxel for previously treated, PD-L1-positive, advanced non-small-cell lung cancer (KEYNOTE-010): a randomised controlled trial. Lancet 2016;387(10027):1540–50.
9. Reck M, Rodríguez-Abreu D, Robinson AG, et al. Updated analysis of KEYNOTE-024: pembrolizumab versus platinum-based chemotherapy for advanced non–small-cell lung cancer with PD-L1 tumor proportion score of 50% or greater. J Clin Oncol 2019; 37(7):537–46.
10. Mok TSK, Wu YL, Kudaba I, et al. Pembrolizumab versus chemotherapy for previously untreated, PD-L1-expressing, locally advanced or metastatic non-small-cell lung cancer (KEYNOTE-042): a randomised, open-label, controlled, phase 3 trial. Lancet 2019;393(10183):1819–30.
11. Leighl NB, Hellmann MD, Hui R, et al. Pembrolizumab in patients with advanced non-small-cell lung cancer (KEYNOTE-001): 3-year results from an open-label, phase 1 study. Lancet Respir Med 2019;7(4):347–57.
12. Borghaei H, Paz-Ares L, Horn L, et al. Nivolumab versus docetaxel in advanced nonsquamous non-small-cell lung cancer. N Engl J Med 2015;373(17): 1627–39.
13. Brahmer J, Reckamp KL, Baas P, et al. Nivolumab versus docetaxel in advanced squamous-cell non-small-cell lung cancer. N Engl J Med 2015;373(2): 123–35.
14. Fehrenbacher L, Spira A, Ballinger M, et al. Atezolizumab versus docetaxel for patients with previously treated non-small-cell lung cancer (POPLAR): a multicentre, open-label, phase 2 randomised controlled trial. Lancet 2016;387(10030):1837–46.
15. Peters S, Gettinger S, Johnson ML, et al. Phase II trial of atezolizumab as first-line or subsequent therapy for patients with programmed death-ligand 1-selected advanced non-small-cell lung cancer (BIRCH). J Clin Oncol 2017;35(24):2781–9.
16. Melendez B, Van Campenhout C, Rorive S, et al. Methods of measurement for tumor mutational burden in tumor tissue. Transl Lung Cancer Res 2018;7(6):661–7.
17. Subbiah V, Kurzrock R. The marriage between genomics and immunotherapy: mismatch meets its match. Oncologist 2019;24(1):1–3.
18. Carbone DP, Reck M, Paz-Ares L, et al. First-line nivolumab in stage IV or recurrent non-small-cell lung cancer. N Engl J Med 2017;376(25):2415–26.
19. Rizvi NA, Hellmann MD, Snyder A, et al. Cancer immunology. Mutational landscape determines sensitivity to PD-1 blockade in non-small cell lung cancer. Science 2015;348(6230):124–8.
20. Hellmann MD, Ciuleanu TE, Pluzanski A, et al. Nivolumab plus Ipilimumab in Lung Cancer with a High Tumor Mutational Burden. N Engl J Med 2018; 378(22):2093–104.
21. Samstein RM, Lee CH, Shoushtari AN, et al. Tumor mutational load predicts survival after immunotherapy across multiple cancer types. Nat Genet 2019;51(2):202–6.
22. Marcus L, Lemery SJ, Keegan P, et al. FDA approval summary: pembrolizumab for the treatment of microsatellite instability-high solid tumors. Clin Cancer Res 2019;25(13):3753–8.
23. Llosa NJ, Cruise M, Tam A, et al. The vigorous immune microenvironment of microsatellite instable colon cancer is balanced by multiple counter-inhibitory checkpoints. Cancer Discov 2015;5(1): 43–51.
24. Le DT, Uram JN, Wang H, et al. PD-1 blockade in tumors with mismatch-repair deficiency. N Engl J Med 2015;372(26):2509–20.
25. Brambilla E, Le Teuff G, Marguet S, et al. Prognostic effect of tumor lymphocytic infiltration in resectable non-small-cell lung cancer. J Clin Oncol 2016; 34(11):1223–30.
26. Lee JS, Ruppin E. Multiomics prediction of response rates to therapies to inhibit programmed cell death 1 and programmed cell death 1 ligand 1. JAMA Oncol 2019. https://doi.org/10.1001/jamaoncol.2019.2311.
27. Dong ZY, Zhang JT, Liu SY, et al. EGFR mutation correlates with uninflamed phenotype and weak immunogenicity, causing impaired response to PD-1

blockade in non-small cell lung cancer. Oncoimmunology 2017;6(11):e1356145.
28. Lisberg A, Cummings A, Goldman JW, et al. A phase II study of pembrolizumab in EGFR-mutant, PD-L1+, tyrosine kinase inhibitor naive patients with advanced NSCLC. J Thorac Oncol 2018;13(8):1138–45.
29. Mazieres J, Drilon A, Lusque A, et al. Immune checkpoint inhibitors for patients with advanced lung cancer and oncogenic driver alterations: results from the IMMUNOTARGET registry. Ann Oncol 2019;30(8):1321–8.
30. Skoulidis F, Goldberg ME, Greenawalt DM, et al. STK11/LKB1 mutations and PD-1 inhibitor resistance in KRAS-mutant lung adenocarcinoma. Cancer Discov 2018;8(7):822–35.
31. Koyama S, Akbay EA, Li YY, et al. STK11/LKB1 deficiency promotes neutrophil recruitment and proinflammatory cytokine production to suppress t-cell activity in the lung tumor microenvironment. Cancer Res 2016;76(5):999–1008.
32. Kitajima S, Ivanova E, Guo S, et al. Suppression of STING associated with LKB1 loss in KRAS-driven lung cancer. Cancer Discov 2019;9(1):34–45.
33. Pan Y, Zheng D, Li Y, et al. Unique distribution of programmed death ligand 1 (PD-L1) expression in East Asian non-small cell lung cancer. J Thorac Dis 2017;9(8):2579–86.
34. Cancer Genome Atlas Research Network. Comprehensive molecular profiling of lung adenocarcinoma. Nature 2014;511(7511):543–50.
35. Rangachari D, VanderLaan PA, Shea M, et al. Correlation between classic driver oncogene mutations in EGFR, ALK, or ROS1 and 22C3-PD-L1 >/=50% expression in lung adenocarcinoma. J Thorac Oncol 2017;12(5):878–83.
36. Gettinger S, Choi J, Hastings K, et al. Impaired HLA class I antigen processing and presentation as a mechanism of acquired resistance to immune checkpoint inhibitors in lung cancer. Cancer Discov 2017;7(12):1420–35.
37. Negrao MV, Lam VK, Reuben A, et al. PD-L1 expression, tumor mutational burden, and cancer gene mutations are stronger predictors of benefit from immune checkpoint blockade than HLA class I genotype in non-small cell lung cancer. J Thorac Oncol 2019;14(6):1021–31.
38. Hu-Lieskovan S, Lisberg A, Zaretsky JM, et al. Tumor characteristics associated with benefit from pembrolizumab in advanced non-small cell lung cancer. Clin Cancer Res 2019;25(16):5061–8.
39. Zhu X, Lang J. Soluble PD-1 and PD-L1: predictive and prognostic significance in cancer. Oncotarget 2017;8(57):97671–82.
40. Gandara DR, Paul SM, Kowanetz M, et al. Blood-based tumor mutational burden as a predictor of clinical benefit in non-small-cell lung cancer patients treated with atezolizumab. Nat Med 2018;24(9):1441–8.
41. Paz-Ares L, Luft A, Vicente D, et al. Pembrolizumab plus chemotherapy for squamous non-small-cell lung cancer. N Engl J Med 2018;379(21):2040–51.

Adjuvant and Neoadjuvant Immunotherapy in Non–small Cell Lung Cancer

Stephen R. Broderick, MD, MPHS

KEYWORDS

• Immunotherapy • Non–small cell lung cancer • Neoadjuvant • Checkpoint blockade

KEY POINTS

- Immunotherapy with immune checkpoint blockade has become a mainstay in the treatment of advanced non–small cell lung cancer.
- The role of checkpoint inhibition in the adjuvant (postresection) setting is unclear and remains under investigation in multiple prospective trials.
- Neoadjuvant checkpoint blockade has been well tolerated and has not led to undue toxicity or surgical morbidity/mortality.
- Early results from phase 1/2 trials suggest promising results, and multiple prospective phase 3 trials, which are powered for survival endpoints, are underway.

Lung cancer accounts for the greatest number of cancer-related mortalities in the United States and worldwide. Non–small cell lung cancer (NSCLC) is the most common lung cancer subtype, comprising 84% of new diagnoses. Despite advances in cross-sectional imaging and the advent of screening programs, most patients are diagnosed with stage IV disease.[1] Surgical resection with curative intent is the mainstay of therapy in early-stage (I–IIIA) NSCLC, with definitive chemoradiation reserved for patients who are deemed unresectable based on tumor characteristics or fitness for surgery. However, despite resection of localized or locoregional disease, 30% to 60% of resected patients will develop metastatic disease.[2] Overall survival in this population remains disappointing with 5-year survival rates of 60% for stage IIA and 36% for patients with stage IIIA disease.[3] The administration of systemic therapy either before (neoadjuvant) or after resection (adjuvant) provides a 5% improvement in overall survival in patients with stage II–IIIA and select patients with large or high-risk IB tumors.[4–6]

The advent of immune checkpoint inhibition has revolutionized treatment strategies in many advanced solid malignancies, including melanoma, head and neck, renal, and lung cancers. The primary immunotherapeutic agents in clinical use modulate the cytotoxic T-lymphocyte-associated protein 4 (CTLA-4; ipilimumab) or programmed cell death protein 1 (PD-1; nivolumab, pembrolizumab, atezolizumab, durvalumab) pathways. CTLA-4 is a glycoprotein expressed on the surface of T cells that binds to costimulatory domains of antigen-presenting cells, inhibiting costimulation of T cells.[7] Programmed cell death protein 1 ligand (PD-L1) is expressed on the surface of tumor cells and binds to the PD-1 receptor on T cells, resulting in downregulation of the T-cell immune response.[8] Inhibition of these regulatory pathways allows for activation of the immune T-cell response to tumors.

CHECKPOINT BLOCKADE IN METASTATIC NON–SMALL CELL LUNG CANCER

Historically, patients with advanced NSCLC were treated with platinum-based cytotoxic

Department of Surgery, Johns Hopkins Medical Institutions, 600 North Wolfe Street, Blalock 240, Baltimore, MD 21287, USA
E-mail address: sbroder7@jhmi.edu
Twitter: @SBroderickMD (S.R.B.)

Thorac Surg Clin 30 (2020) 215–220
https://doi.org/10.1016/j.thorsurg.2020.01.001
1547-4127/20/

chemotherapy, with a median survival of 8 to 12 months.[9] Data from the CHECKMATE-017, CHECKMATE-057, KEYNOTE-010, and POPLAR/OAK studies published in 2015 to 2017 provided the basis for the use of nivolumab (PD-1), pembrolizumab (PD-L1), and atezolizumab (PD-L1) as single-agent therapies in patients previously treated for NSCLC with progression of disease.[10–14]

Subsequent studies have demonstrated substantial improvements in overall survival with checkpoint blockade in the first-line setting either alone or in combination with chemotherapy. KEYNOTE-024 was a randomized trial of first-line pembrolizumab versus platinum doublet chemotherapy in patients whose tumors expressed high levels of PD-L1 on the cell surface (PD-L1 Tumor Proportion Score [TPS] ≥50%). Results demonstrated a median survival of 30 months with pembrolizumab compared with 14.2 months with platinum doublet, along with a favorable toxicity profile.[15] The KEYNOTE-189 trial then demonstrated a similar doubling of survival for patients receiving pembrolizumab in conjunction with chemotherapy compared with chemotherapy alone.[16] Additional studies have now demonstrated similar increased efficacy of anti–PD-1/PD-L1 therapy with chemotherapy in both squamous and nonsquamous NSCLC.[17,18] Thus, anti–PD-1/PD-L1 therapy has become a mainstay in the treatment of metastatic NSCLC.

CHECKPOINT BLOCKADE IN LOCOREGIONAL NON–SMALL CELL LUNG CANCER

The efficacy of immune checkpoint blockade in advanced NSCLC has naturally stimulated interest in studying the application of these agents in earlier-stage disease. In patients with unresectable stage III NSCLC, concurrent chemoradiotherapy is standard-of-care treatment. However, long-term outcomes remain poor, with 5-year survival of 15%.[19] The PACIFIC trial was a prospective randomized trial in which patients with locally advanced, unresectable stage III NSCLC were randomized to consolidation therapy with durvalumab (anti–PD-L1) for up to 1 year or placebo. Results demonstrated a median progression-free survival of 17.2 months in the durvalumab group compared with 5.6 months with placebo.[20] This study resulted in the approval of durvalumab as consolidation therapy following concurrent chemoradiation in unresectable stage III NSCLC.

ADJUVANT CHECKPOINT BLOCKADE

The role of immune checkpoint blockade in the adjuvant (postresection) setting is less defined and has not demonstrated meaningful clinical benefit as yet in resected NSCLC. It has, however, shown a significant increase in survival as adjuvant therapy in stage III melanoma with ipilimumab[21] and more recently stage III–IV melanoma with nivolumab.[22]

For patients with resected stage IB–IIIA NSCLC, 4 large phase 3 studies of adjuvant PD-1/PD-L1 blockade are ongoing (**Table 1**). The ANVIL study (NCT02595944) compares 1 year of nivolumab following surgery with or without adjuvant cytotoxic chemotherapy with observation alone. Primary endpoints for this study are disease-free survival and overall survival. IMpower-010 (NCT02486718) is a phase 3 study comparing 16 cycles of atezolizumab to best supportive care after resection and adjuvant chemotherapy with primary endpoint of disease-free survival. The PEARLS (NCT02504372) study compares 1 year of pembrolizumab to observation following surgery with or without standard adjuvant chemotherapy with primary endpoint of disease-free survival. The National Cancer Institute of Canada (NCT02273375) is investigating durvalumab

Table 1
Ongoing clinical trials to evaluate the efficacy of adjuvant checkpoint blockade in resected non–small cell lung cancer

Trial	Phase	Stage	Adjuvant Therapy	Primary Endpoint(s)
ANVIL (NCT02595944)	3	IB[a]–IIIA	Nivolumab + chemotherapy	OS DFS
IMpower010 (NCT02486718)	3	IB[a]–IIIA	Atezolizumab + chemotherapy	DFS
PEARLS/KEYNOTE-091 (NCT02504372)	3	IB[a]–IIIA	Pembrolizumab vs placebo with or without chemotherapy	DFS
NCT02273375	3	IB[a]–IIIB[b]	Durvalumab vs placebo with or without chemotherapy	DFS

Abbreviations: DFS, disease-free survival; OS, overall survival.
[a] IB tumors ≥4 cm.
[b] T3N2M0.

Table 2
Ongoing clinical trials to evaluate the safety, feasibility, and efficacy of neoadjuvant checkpoint blockade in combination with chemotherapy

Trial	Phase	Stage	Neoadjuvant Therapy	Primary Endpoint(s)
CHECKMATE-816 (NCT02998528)	3	IB[a]–IIIA	Chemotherapy vs chemotherapy + nivolumab	EFS pCR
IMPOWER-030 (NCT03456063)	3	IB[a]–IIIA	Chemotherapy + atezolizumab vs chemotherapy + placebo	MPR EFS
KEYNOTE-671 (NCT03425643)	3	II–IIIB[b]	Chemotherapy + pembrolizumab vs chemotherapy	EFS OS
NCT03800134	3	II–IIIB[b]	Chemotherapy + durvalumab vs chemotherapy + placebo	MPR

Abbreviations: EFS, event-free survival; pCR, pathologic complete response.
[a] IB tumors ≥4 cm.
[b] T3N2M0.

versus placebo in the adjuvant setting with primary endpoint of disease-free survival. Estimated completion dates for all of the adjuvant trials are 2024 to 2027. Thus, the role of PD-1/PD-L1 blockade in the adjuvant setting will likely remain unclear for some time. However, results of these studies may have a substantial impact on practice for patients with resected locoregional NSCLC.

RATIONALE FOR NEOADJUVANT CHECKPOINT BLOCKADE

There are several advantages, both conceptual and practical, to the administration of immune checkpoint inhibitors in the neoadjuvant setting. With neoadjuvant administration, the intact tumor may serve as a source for antigen-specific T-cell immunity with a diverse antigen load. Resection of the tumor and pathologic analysis after treatment also allow for an early assessment of treatment response in individual patients, allowing for potential to adjust systemic therapy based on pathologic response. Finally, neoadjuvant protocols provide a unique platform for correlative basic and translational investigations.[23]

Some of the above advantages are highlighted by a murine model of triple-negative breast cancer in which investigators compared neoadjuvant and adjuvant administration of anti–PD-1/anti-CD137 combination therapy. Mice treated with the drug before surgery demonstrated a 40% long-term survival compared with 0% in the adjuvant group. In addition, the neoadjuvant group showed an increase in tumor-specific $CD8^+$ T cells that was not seen in the adjuvant group, suggesting that treatment with the tumor in situ prompted a more robust T-cell response.[24] Application of neoadjuvant PD-1/PD-L1 blockade has suggested safety, feasibility, and efficacy in solid tumors other than NSCLC, including melanoma (OpACIN), triple-negative breast cancer (KEYNOTE-173), and urothelial carcinomas.[25–27]

EXISTING EVIDENCE FOR NEOADJUVANT CHECKPOINT BLOCKADE

Among the first studies of neoadjuvant checkpoint inhibition in early-stage NSCLC was a study by Forde and colleagues.[28] This study was a phase 2 study designed to evaluate the safety and feasibility of administration of 2 doses of nivolumab over 4 weeks before surgery in patients with stage I–IIIA resectable NSCLC. Twenty-one patients were enrolled in the study and received nivolumab preoperatively. The treatment was well tolerated, and there were no delays to planned resection. Toxicity was noted in 5 of 21 patients, with grade 3 or higher toxicity in only 1 patient with pneumonia. Twenty of 21 patients underwent resection, with 1 patient deemed unresectable at the time of surgery because of tracheal invasion. Most patients (75%) underwent lobectomy, and most resections (70%) were completed via an open approach. Analysis of surgical outcomes demonstrated no mortalities and a morbidity profile consistent with prior studies of neoadjuvant chemotherapy or chemoradiotherapy.[29] Resection specimens showed a major pathologic response rate (≤10 residual viable tumor) of 45% with 2 (10%) complete pathologic responses. Sixteen of 20 resected patients were alive without recurrence at 1 year after resection, and median disease-free and overall survival have not yet been reached.

There were several additional important clinical and translational findings reported from this study. Patients underwent repeat imaging after treatment with nivolumab, before resection. Notably, post-treatment imaging findings did not correlate with pathologic response. Although 45% of patients demonstrated major pathologic response (MPR), the vast majority (85%) of patients had stable radiographic disease by RECIST criteria, with 2 (10%) demonstrating partial response and 1 (5%) demonstrating progression. This finding is likely secondary to T-cell infiltration of the primary tumor and is an important phenomenon for surgeons considering resection for patients along a neoadjuvant immunotherapy paradigm. Anecdotally, surgeons noted enlargement of lymph nodes that did not correlate with pathologic nodal involvement as well as inflammation or fibrosis in the pulmonary hilum.

Contrary to what has been demonstrated in advanced disease, whereby PD-L1 expression was correlated with clinical response to single-agent checkpoint inhibition,[15] in the Forde study, pathologic response did not correlate with PD-L1 expression on pretreatment tumor biopsy. Tumor mutation burden from whole-exome sequencing of pretreatment biopsies was shown to correlate with pathologic response. Finally, analysis of peripheral blood identified an expansion of tumor-specific T cells after anti–PD-1 therapy. This population of T cells decreased following resection but remained detectable, suggesting the possibility of a durable antitumor immunity.

A second analysis of single-agent neoadjuvant checkpoint inhibitor (LCMC-3, NCT02927301) was presented in abstract form at the American Society of Clinical Oncology (ASCO) 2019 annual meeting.[29] This abstract was an interim analysis of the first 101 of a planned 180 patients who received 2 doses of atezolizumab before resection. This analysis demonstrated similar acceptable perioperative outcomes with 1 perioperative mortality. Ninety of 101 patients underwent resection; 10 patients demonstrated progression of disease during neoadjuvant therapy, and 1 patient was found to be unresectable at exploration. MPR rate was 18% with 6 complete pathologic responses. Analysis of imaging studies demonstrated a similar lack of concordance with radiographic and pathologic results as in the Forde study. PD-L1 staining by TPS (≥50%) correlated with response, whereas tumor mutation burden did not in this analysis.

Results of the multicenter NADIM (NCT03081689) (*Neoad*juvant *Im*munotherapy) study have shown the most promising response data to date.[30] This study is a phase 2 trial of neoadjuvant carboplatin/paclitaxel combined with 3 cycles of nivolumab followed by adjuvant nivolumab for 1 year in patients with stage IIIA NSCLC. At the time of last update, 41 of 46 patients had undergone surgery. No patients experienced a delay to surgery or were withdrawn because of toxicity or progression during neoadjuvant therapy. The primary endpoint for NADIM is progression-free survival; however, a remarkable 34 of 41 (83%) patients achieved major pathologic response with 24 of 41 (71%) achieving complete pathologic response. As seen in other neoadjuvant studies, radiographic response did not correlate with pathologic response.

Results of the phase 2 NEOSTAR (NCT03158129) were presented at ASCO in 2019.[31] This study randomized patients with resectable stage I–III NSCLC to neoadjuvant therapy with nivolumab or nivolumab + ipilimumab before resection. The rationale for the addition of ipilimumab was provided by the results of the CHECKMATE-012 trial, which demonstrated an improvement in progression-free survival in patients treated with combined PD-1 (nivolumab) and CTLA-4 (ipilimumab) blockade.[32] Forty-four patients were randomized: 23 to nivolumab only, 21 to nivolumab + ipilimumab. Seven patients (5 in nivolumab + ipilimumab arm) did not undergo planned resection. Overall MPR rate was 25% (17% in the nivolumab only arm; 33% in the nivolumab + ipilimumab arm). This study also identified higher response rates in tumors with a high proportion of PD-L1 expression. Further details regarding the LCMC-3, NEOSTAR, and NADIM trials will be forthcoming with final analyses and publication.

ONGOING STUDIES EXAMINING NEOADJUVANT CHECKPOINT BLOCKADE

Although many phase 2 studies continue to accrue, encouraging results from these studies have led to substantial enthusiasm to conduct phase 3 trials. Studies to date have used MPR rate as a surrogate endpoint, and there is evidence correlating MPR with survival.[33] Several phase 3 studies of neoadjuvant checkpoint blockade are currently accruing (**Table 2**), many of which are powered to evaluate survival endpoints. CHECKMATE-816 (NCT02998528) has randomized 350 patients with stage IB (≥4 cm) to IIIA NSCLC to platinum-based chemotherapy plus nivolumab or chemotherapy alone. A third arm of the study in which patients received nivolumab plus ipilimumab has been discontinued. This trial has recently completed accrual. Primary endpoints are pathologic complete response and event-free survival. IMPOWER-030 (NCT03456063) evaluates neoadjuvant platinum doublet chemotherapy in conjunction with either atezolizumab or placebo in patients with stage II or IIIA NSCLC. Select patients with stage IIIB disease are also eligible. This study has a target enrollment of 374 patients and primary endpoints are MPR and event-free survival. KEYNOTE-671 (NCT03425643) is another placebo-controlled randomized trial evaluating neoadjuvant chemotherapy with or without pembrolizumab followed by adjuvant chemotherapy. Target enrollment for this trial is 786 patients and is powered for event-free and overall survival comparisons. NCT03800134 is a similar trial evaluating chemotherapy with durvalumab compared with chemotherapy with placebo in patients with resectable stage IIA–IIIB NSCLC. Target enrollment is 300 patients, and primary endpoint is MPR.

NEOADJUVANT IMMUNORADIATION

A secondary analysis of the phase 1 KEYNOTE-001 study suggested improved progression-free and overall survival in patients treated with pembrolizumab who had previously received radiotherapy.[34,35] Safety and efficacy of combination checkpoint blockade and radiotherapy are under investigation in several studies. In a pilot study at Johns Hopkins University, patients with stage IIIA NSCLC resectable by lobectomy receive durvalumab or durvalumab plus tremelimumab with standard radiation therapy (45 Gy in 25 fractions) before resection (NCT03237377). The primary outcomes of this study are safety and feasibility. A second trial at Weill Cornell (NCT02904954) randomizes patients with resectable stage II–III NSCLC to 2 doses of neoadjuvant durvalumab with or without concurrent nonablative radiotherapy (8 Gy $\times$ 4 doses) with primary outcome of disease-free survival. A separate Kelly Fitzgerald and Charles B. Simone's article, "Combining Immunotherapy with Radiation Therapy in Non-small Cell Lung Cancer," in this issue is dedicated to the combination of immunotherapy and radiation.

SUMMARY AND FUTURE DIRECTIONS

Therapies that prevent recurrence of early-stage, resected NSCLC are urgently needed. Despite surgical resection, a proportion of patients with stage I and many patients with locally advanced disease will develop recurrent NSCLC. Early results from studies of neoadjuvant administration of checkpoint inhibitors show promising clinical results and offer a window for scientific analyses of the antitumor immune response. Phase 2 studies suggest safety and feasibility of administration of checkpoint inhibitors with or without chemotherapy in the preoperative setting with acceptable toxicity and perioperative morbidity and mortality. Results of phase 3 studies with survival endpoints may significantly alter treatment strategies for patients with locally advanced NSCLC.

Despite the rapid advances in the field made over the past several years, significant areas of investigation remain, including optimal neoadjuvant regimens, timing of resection after treatment, potential benefit of radiotherapy, and the impact of adjuvant therapy after resection. Surgeon participation in the planning and execution of neoadjuvant trials is critical because optimal strategies for patients with locoregional NSCLC continue to evolve.

DISCLOSURE

Dr S.R. Broderick serves as a consultant for Bristol-Myers Squibb.

REFERENCES

1. Siegel RL, Miller KD, Jemal A. Cancer Statistics 2017. CA Cancer J Clin 2017;67:7–30.
2. Boyd JA, Hubbs JL, Kim DW, et al. Timing of local and distant failure in resected lung cancer: implications for reported rates of local failure. J Thorac Oncol 2010;5:211–4.
3. Goldstraw P, Chansky K, Crowley J, et al. The IASLC lung cancer staging project: proposals for revision of the TNM stage groupings in the forthcoming (eighth) edition of the TNM classification of lung cancer. J Thorac Oncol 2016;11:39–51.
4. Arriagada R, Bergman B, Dunant A, et al. Cisplatin-based adjuvant chemotherapy in patients with completely resected non-small cell lung cancer. N Engl J Med 2004;350:351–60.
5. Butts CA, Ding K, Seymour L, et al. Randomized phase III trial of vinorelbine plus cisplatin compared with observation in completely resected stage IB and II non-small cell lung cancer: updated survival analysis of JBR-10. J Clin Oncol 2010;28:29–34.
6. Scagliotti GV, Fossati R, Torri V, et al. Randomized study of adjuvant chemotherapy for completely resected stage I, II, or IIIA non-small-cell lung cancer. J Natl Cancer Inst 2003;95:1453–61.
7. Walker LS, Sansom DM. The emerging role of CTLA4 as a cell-extrinsic regulator of T cell responses. Nat Rev Immunol 2011;11:852–63.
8. Keir ME, Butte MJ, Freeman GJ, et al. PD-1 and its ligands in tolerance and immunity. Annu Rev Immunol 2008;26:677–704.
9. Socinski MA, Bondarenko I, Karaseva NA, et al. Weekly nab-paclitaxel in combination with carboplatin versus solvent-based paclitaxel plus carboplatin as first-line therapy in patients with advanced non-small-cell lung cancer: final results of a phase III trial. J Clin Oncol 2012;30:2055–62.
10. Brahmer J, Reckamp KL, Baas P, et al. Nivolumab versus docetaxel in advanced squamous-cell non-small-cell lung cancer. N Engl J Med 2015;373:1627–39.
11. Borghaei H, Paz-Ares L, Horn L, et al. Nivolumab versus docetaxel in advanced nonsquamous non-small-cell lung cancer. N Engl J Med 2015;373:123–35.

12. Herbst RS, Baas P, Kim DW, et al. Pembrolizumab versus docetaxel for previously treated PD-L1-positive, advanced non-small-cell lung cancer (KEYNOTE-010): a randomised controlled trial. Lancet 2016;387:1540–50.
13. Fehrenbacher L, Spira A, Ballinger M, et al. Atezolizumab versus docetaxel for patients with previously treated non-small-cell lung cancer (POPLAR): a multicentre, open-label, phase 2 randomised controlled trial. Lancet 2016;387:1837–46.
14. Rittmeyer A, Barlesi F, Waterkamp D, et al. Atezolizumab versus docetaxel in patients with previously treated non-small-cell lung cancer (OAK): a phase 3, open-label, multicenter randomised controlled trial. Lancet 2017;389:255–65.
15. Reck M, Rodriquez-Abreu D, Robinson AG, et al. Pembrolizumab versus chemotherapy for PD-L1 positive non-small-cell lung cancer. N Engl J Med 2016;375:1823–33.
16. Gandhi L, Rodrigues-Abreu D, Gadgeel S, et al. Pembrolizumab plus chemotherapy in metastatic non-small-cell lung cancer. N Engl J Med 2018; 378:2078–92.
17. Langer CJ, Gadgeel SM, Borghaei H, et al. Carboplatin and pemetrexed with or without pembrolizumab for advanced, non-squamous non-small-cell lung cancer: a randomised, phase 2 cohort of the open-label KEYNOTE-021 study. Lancet Oncol 2016;17:1497–508.
18. Socinski MA, Jotte RM, Cappuzzo F, et al. Atezolizumab for first-line treatment of metastatic non-squamous NSCLC. N Engl J Med 2018;378:2280–301.
19. Auperin A, Le Pechoux C, Rolland E, et al. Meta-analysis of concomitant versus sequential radiochemotherapy in locally advanced non-small-cell lung cancer. J Clin Oncol 2010;28:2181–90.
20. Antonia SJ, Villegas A, Daniel D, et al. Durvalumab after chemoradiotherapy in stage III non-small-cell lung cancer. N Engl J Med 2017;377:1919–29.
21. Eggermont AM, Chiarion-Sileni V, Grob JJ, et al. Adjuvant ipilimumab versus placebo after complete resection of high-risk stage III melanoma (EORTC 18071): a randomised, double-blind, phase 3 trial. Lancet Oncol 2015;16:522–30.
22. Weber J, Mandala M, Del Vecchio M, et al. Adjuvant nivolumab versus ipilimumab in resected stage III or IV melanoma. N Engl J Med 2017;377:1824–35.
23. Owen D, Chaft J. Immunotherapy in surgically resectable non-small-cell lung cancer. J Thorac Dis 2018;10(suppl 3):S404–11.
24. Liu J, Blake SJ, Yong MC, et al. Improved efficacy of neoadjuvant compared to adjuvant immunotherapy to eradicate metastatic disease. Cancer Discov 2016;6:1382–99.
25. Rozeman EA, Blank CU, VanAkkooi A, et al. Neoadjuvant ipilimumab + nivolumab (IPI + NIVO) in palpable stage III melanoma: updated data from the OpACIN trial and first immunological analyses. J Clin Oncol 2017;35(suppl 15):9586.
26. Schmid P, Park YH, Munoz-Couselo E, et al. Pembrolizumab (pembro) + chemotherapy (chemo) as neoadjuvant treatment for triple negative breast cancer (TNBC): preliminary results from KEYNOTE-173. J Clin Oncol 2017;35(suppl 15):556.
27. Carthon BC, Wolchok JD, Yuan J, et al. Preoperative CTLA-4 blockade: tolerability and immune monitoring in the setting of a presurgical clinical trial. Clin Cancer Res 2010;16:2861–71.
28. Forde PM, Chaft JE, William WN, et al. Neoadjuvant PD-1 blockade in resectable lung cancer. N Engl J Med 2018;378:1976–86.
29. Bott MJ, Yang SC, Park BJ, et al. Initial results of pulmonary resection after neoadjuvant nivolumab in patients with resectable non-small cell lung cancer. J Thorac Cardiovasc Surg 2019;158:269–76.
30. Rusch V, Chaft JE, Johnson B, et al. Neoadjuvant atezolizumab in resectable non-small-cell lung cancer (NSCLC): initial results from a multicenter study (LCMC3). Abstract presented at American Society of Clinical Oncology Annual Meeting. Chicago, IL, June 3, 2018.
31. Provencio-Pulla M, Nadal-Alforja E, Cobo M, et al. Neoadjuvant chemo/immunotherapy for the treatment of stage IIIA resectable non-small cell lung cancer (NSCLC): a phase II multicenter exploratory study–final data of patients who underwent surgical resection. Abstract presented at American Society of Clinical Oncology Annual Meeting. Chicago, IL, June 2, 2019.
32. Cascone T, William WN, Weissferdt A, et al. Neoadjuvant nivolumab (N) or nivolumab plus ipilimumab (NI) for resectable non-small cell lung cancer (NSCLC): clinical results from the NEOSTAR study. J Clin Oncol 2019;37(15_suppl):8504 [abstract].
33. Hellman MD, Ciuleanu TE, Pluzanski A, et al. Nivolumab plus ipilimumab in lung cancer with a high tumor mutational burden. N Engl J Med 2018;378: 2093–104.
34. Hellmann MD, Chaft JE, William WN, et al. Pathological response after neoadjuvant chemotherapy in resectable non-small-cell lung cancers: proposal for the use of major pathological response as a surrogate endpoint. Lancet Oncol 2014;15:e42–50.
35. Shaverdian N, Lisberg AE, Bornazyan K, et al. Previous radiotherapy and the clinical activity and toxicity of pembrolizumab in the treatment of non-small-cell lung cancer: a secondary analysis of the KEYNOTE-001 phase 1 trial. Lancet Oncol 2017;18:895–903.

Combining Immunotherapy with Radiation Therapy in Non–Small Cell Lung Cancer

Kelly Fitzgerald, MD, PhD[a], Charles B. Simone II, MD[a,b,*]

KEYWORDS

- Immunotherapy • Immune checkpoint inhibitors • Radiation therapy • Lung cancer
- Systemic therapy

KEY POINTS

- The efficacy of current treatment approaches with cytotoxic chemotherapy for lung cancer is limited.
- Immune checkpoint inhibitors have recently been demonstrated to improve survival in metastatic and locally advanced lung cancer.
- Radiation therapy has been shown to be immunostimulatory and may enhance the efficacy of immunotherapy.
- Numerous trials combining radiation therapy and immunotherapy are ongoing in early-stage, locally advanced, and metastatic non–small cell lung cancer.

INTRODUCTION

Lung cancer is the second most common cancer in men and women in the United States and the leading cause of cancer death in both sexes.[1] Non–small cell histology represents the largest subtype and comprises approximately 85% of all lung cancers. Broad treatment paradigms for non–small cell lung cancer (NSCLC) include surgical resection or stereotactic body radiation therapy (SBRT) for early-stage disease, surgery, and chemotherapy with or without radiotherapy or definitive chemoradiation for locally advanced disease, and various systemic therapies for metastatic disease.[2] These traditional therapies offer limited long-term disease control, with historical 5-year survival rates of 5% for patients presenting with stage IV disease. Even early-stage disease carries a notable risk of developing metastases after initial surgical or radiosurgical management, with 2-year rates of nodal failure of 10% to 15% and distant failure of ~15% to 20%.[3] Thus, there is a significant unmet need for improved treatments across all stages of this cancer.

In the past decade, T-cell checkpoint blockade has emerged as a routine treatment for numerous solid tumors, including NSCLC.[4] The use of these drugs in NSCLC was first established in the second-line metastatic setting,[5–8] and their role has now been extended to treating first-line metastatic[9] and even locally advanced disease.[10] Intense interest is now focused on incorporating checkpoint blockade into treatment of even earlier

Funding: None.

[a] Department of Radiation Oncology, Memorial Sloan Kettering Cancer Center, 1275 First Avenue, Mezzanine Level, New York, NY 10065, USA; [b] New York Proton Center, 225 East 126th Street, New York, NY 10035, USA
* Corresponding author. New York Proton Center, 225 East 126th Street, New York, NY 10035.
E-mail address: csimone@nyproton.com

Thorac Surg Clin 30 (2020) 221–239
https://doi.org/10.1016/j.thorsurg.2020.01.002
1547-4127/20/

stage disease in optimal combination with local therapies such as surgery or radiation therapy (RT).

RADIATION IN NON–SMALL CELL LUNG CANCER

RT is a key treatment modality for NSCLC in the definitive setting, particularly in patients who are medically unfit for surgery. Because of the frequent occurrence of medical comorbidities (including smoking-induced chronic obstructive pulmonary disease and heart disease) in the elderly and smoker population most likely to develop lung cancer, a significant percentage of patients can tolerate only noninvasive therapies.

In early disease, highly conformal, hypofractionated RT is the standard of care for medically inoperable patients, is an emerging treatment option for operable patients, and offers local control rates of approximately 90% to 95%, similar to lobectomy.[11–13] This type of radiation, known as either SBRT or stereotactic ablative body radiation (SABR), is delivered most commonly in 1 to 5 fractions with a high dose of radiation per fraction.[14] Conventionally fractionated radiation regimens delivered over several weeks are used in more advanced node-positive disease and are better tolerated by central structures, such as the esophagus, heart, and central airway compared with SBRT. In locally advanced disease, radiation can be used in the neoadjuvant[15,16] or adjuvant[17] setting, but it is more commonly used as a definitive treatment for unresectable patients or those who are more frail and medically inoperable.[18] Platinum-based chemotherapy acts as a radiosensitizer, and a metaanalysis of several trials demonstrated improved overall survival (OS) with concurrent chemotherapy compared with sequential chemotherapy and radiation.[19]

Traditionally, the role of RT in the setting of metastatic NSCLC was mainly one of palliation for symptoms like pain, hemoptysis, or dyspnea.[20,21] New evidence suggests that radiation can improve survival in limited oligometastatic disease. Gomez and colleagues[22] reported on a phase 2 clinical trial in which patients with stage IV NSCLC without progression after 3 months of first-line therapy were randomized to receive local consolidative therapy (radiation or surgery) to 3 or fewer metastases versus observation/maintenance therapy. Those treated with local therapy to all metastases saw their OS more than double compared with controls (median OS of 41.2 months vs 17.0 months). This study is supported by the similar phase 2 SABR-COMET trial that randomized patients with multiple cancer subtypes, including NSCLC, to observation/maintenance therapy versus radiation to up to 5 metastases.[23] Patients who received radiation in the SABR-COMET study similarly had nearly a doubling of OS. Phase 3 trials (NRG Oncology LU002) are ongoing to confirm these promising results.

IMMUNE CHECKPOINT BLOCKADE

Immune checkpoint blockade (ICB) drugs remove molecular brakes on T-cell activation, lowering the threshold for immunologic recognition and rejection of cancer. Food and Drug Administration–approved drugs within this therapeutic class include monoclonal antibodies that inhibit cytotoxic T-lymphocyte-associated protein 4 (CTLA-4), programmed cell death protein 1 (PD-1), or programmed cell death protein 1 ligand (PD-L1). The PD-1 inhibitors pembrolizumab, nivolumab are approved for use in metastatic NSCLC,[5–8] and the PD-L1 inhibitor atezolizumab is also approved in the first-line metastatic setting.[8] Durvalumab, which also targets PD-L1, is approved as consolidative therapy following definitive chemoradiation for locally advanced, unresectable NSCLC.[10]

Although these agents have significantly improved median survival compared with older therapies, most patients do not respond to ICB treatment, and a portion of patients who initially respond eventually progress. The former scenario represents primary or intrinsic resistance to ICB, whereas the latter indicates secondary or acquired resistance. Although research has identified tumor characteristics that are predictive of response to immunotherapy, including tumor mutational burden, PD-L1 expression levels, and T-cell infiltration into the tumor, much remains to be elucidated regarding mechanisms of resistance.[24]

THE INTERSECTION OF RADIATION AND IMMUNOTHERAPY

RT, in addition to being highly effective in local tumor control, has demonstrated clear immunomodulatory effects in both preclinical and clinical studies. In mice, radiation to a tumor can act as an in situ vaccine, causing locoregional antigen-presenting cells to increase their uptake and display of cancer neoantigens (mutated peptides that differ from normal proteins and can be recognized as foreign by the immune system). Radiation also creates a proinflammatory cytokine context for this presentation through release of cytosolic DNA and stimulation of the type I interferon pathway. Cytotoxic T cells can then be activated against non–self-antigens and can traffic to sites of tumor.[25]

The most dramatic manifestation of radiation-induced systemic immune activation is termed the abscopal effect, in which radiation to 1 metastatic site induces antitumor responses in distant, nonirradiated sites. This rare effect has been reported in the literature since the 1950s with radiation alone. In 2012, a fascinating case was reported by Postow and colleagues,[26] in which a patient with metastatic melanoma receiving anti-CTLA-4 therapy was treated with radiation to a paraspinal mass, and subsequently the patient achieved reduction not only of the irradiated lesion but also of out-of-field splenic and pulmonary lesions. Such abscopal effects have been infrequently reported for thoracic tumors with RT alone, with RT combined with ICB, and with RT combined with other types of immune therapy, such as immunogene therapy.[27] A 2019 literature review identified 6 case reports in NSCLC that have been published with evidence of an abscopal effect from RT, 4 of which also involved treatment with ICB.[28]

Natural checks and balances within the immune system can counteract the immunostimulatory effects of radiation. For instance, in several mouse models of cancer (breast, colon, melanoma), tumor PD-L1 expression has been shown to increase after radiation, reflecting enhanced resistance to T-cell–mediated killing.[29,30] Likewise, radiation also causes an increase in $CD8^+$ T-cell expression of the cognate receptor PD-1 and the transcription factor Eomes; these markers are associated with an exhausted phenotype that is unable to eliminate tumor cells.[29] In a study of 45 patients with locally advanced NSCLC treated with neoadjuvant chemoradiation followed by surgery, PD-L1 expression on tumor cells significantly decreased or stayed the same in most patients after chemoradiation.[31] The discrepancy of these findings with the mouse data may be due to the use of concurrent chemotherapy along with RT or with the timing of the post-RT analysis. A median of 32 days elapsed between the end of chemoradiation and surgery, whereas in the mouse models, PD-L1 expression was found to peak 3 days after the final fraction of RT. Of note, however, median OS was significantly worse for the few patients in which PD-L1 expression increased compared with those in whom PD-L1 levels decreased. Further confirmation of the preclinical findings in humans has been challenging because of the need to obtain paired pretreatment and posttreatment lung biopsies, although translational clinical trials with this goal are actively recruiting.

Whether the effects are synergistic or merely additive, there is sound mechanistic rationale for integrating RT with ICB[32–34] (**Box 1**). The remainder of this article reviews published clinical data on this combination in all stages of NSCLC, and it highlights ongoing trials of particular interest.

RADIATION AND IMMUNOTHERAPY IN METASTATIC NON–SMALL CELL LUNG CANCER

ICB was first investigated for efficacy against NSCLC in the metastatic setting, where RT most typically plays only a palliative role. A secondary analysis of the phase 1 KEYNOTE 001 trial examined patients with metastatic NSCLC who received RT before their first dose of pembrolizumab (43 of 97 patients). This analysis demonstrated improved median OS (10.7 vs 5.3 months) and progression-free survival (PFS) in patients in which pembrolizumab followed RT.[35] In addition, a large, single-institution retrospective study showed a positive correlation between OS and receiving ICB for more than 30 days before radiation compared with receiving it for less than 30 days or up to 30 days after RT.[36]

Several small trials then began to prospectively investigate the frequency of the abscopal effect with combined RT and ICB. An early trial tested the anti-CTLA-4 antibody ipilimumab and SBRT in patients with a variety of solid malignancies; 8 of 35 patients enrolled had NSCLC.[37] SBRT was directed to either a single lung or liver lesion and was administered either concurrently or sequentially (during cycle 2) with ipilimumab. Ten percent of patients experienced a partial response (excluding the irradiated lesion), and 23% had either a partial response or stable disease lasting $\geq$6 months. Radiation of liver lesions compared with lung lesions caused an increase in $CD8^+$ T cells with expression of inducible T-cell costimulator, glucocorticoid-induced tumor necrosis factor

Box 1
Potential mechanisms of radiation-induced immunostimulation

1. Increased expression of neoantigens
2. Increased release of proinflammatory signals (danger-associated molecular patterns, cytokines)
3. Increased priming of dendritic cells and enhanced cross-presentation of neoantigens
4. Increased infiltration of $CD8^+$ T cells into tumors and/or stimulation of preexisting tumor-infiltrating lymphocytes

receptor, and lymphocyte activation gene 3. Another single-arm trial exclusively in metastatic NSCLC combined ipilimumab with concurrent SBRT to 6 Gy × 5 or 8 Gy × 3 to a single site of disease.[38] This trial yielded an objective response rate of 18%, with 2 complete responses and 5 partial responses. When stable disease was also considered, 31% of patients derived clinical benefit. T-cell clonal expansion pretreatment and posttreatment was analyzed and yielded an interesting mechanistic finding in 1 patient who experienced a complete response. In this patient, an expanded population of T cells in the peripheral blood and tumor was matched to a specific mutated protein (karyopherin A2), which was shown to be upregulated by RT. These results are particularly encouraging when in context with the relative lack of efficacy seen with anti-CTLA-4 antibodies in metastatic NSCLC alone or in combination with chemotherapy.[39]

Data from larger and randomized trials assessing the abscopal response have now begun to mature. The recently published phase 2 PEMBRO RT trial randomized 76 patients to pembrolizumab with or without SBRT given to 1 metastatic site before ICB.[40] Patients had to have at least 2 metastases (no maximum number dictated, average number per patient not reported) and be progressing after chemotherapy. No prior immunotherapy or RT within the last 6 months was allowed. More than half (58%) of patients on the experimental arm received SBRT to an intrathoracic site. The primary endpoint was 50% overall response rate (ORR) as determined by an independent reviewer according to RECIST criteria (version 1.1) and excluding the irradiated lesion. The addition of SBRT doubled the 12-week ORR (from 18% to 36%) but did not meet the prespecified endpoint. Nonetheless, the results are considered promising, and a larger phase 2/3 trial with the same design is expected to follow.

In contrast, a similar phase 1/2 study (NCT02444741) in which 103 patients with metastatic NSCLC were randomized to pembrolizumab with or without RT to a lung lesion did not show a significant out-of-field response rate benefit with addition of radiotherapy.[41] Radiation on this trial could be either SBRT (if the lesion was smaller and in a more favorable location) or conventional RT to 45 Gy in 15 fractions. In an exploratory analysis, however, median PFS was improved for those who received SBRT and pembrolizumab compared with those who received conventional RT and pembrolizumab. The divergent results from these 2 trials highlight the importance of dose and fractionation as variables in stimulating an antitumor immune response.

Other trials have focused on the oligometastatic space, integrating data showing the promise of durable local control by irradiating all sites of metastatic disease with the improved systemic control offered by ICB. A single-arm phase 2 trial was recently reported in *JAMA Oncology* that treated patients with local therapy (surgery or RT) to all sites of disease with the addition of pembrolizumab 4 to 12 weeks later.[42] The study group consisted of 51 patients with metastatic NSCLC and 4 or fewer sites of disease. Median PFS from the start of local therapy was 19.1 months, significantly improved over historical controls of 6.6 months. At the reported median follow-up of 25 months, survival at 1 year was a very promising at 90.9%, and additional follow-up is needed to further assess OS in this cohort.

Although current opinion on the optimal timing is far from uniform,[43] several ongoing studies are designed to investigate the question of optimal timing of RT with respect to immunotherapy (**Table 1**). One such trial from University of California, Davis (NCT02400814) is a nonrandomized parallel-assignment trial in which 45 patients are assigned to 1 of 3 regimens: atezolizumab and SBRT both started on day 1 of cycle 1 (concurrent arm), atezolizumab followed by SBRT on day 1 of cycle 3 (induction arm), or SBRT followed by atezolizumab (sequential arm). The SABRseq trial will divide 32 patients between a regimen of SBRT followed by pembrolizumab or pembrolizumab followed by SBRT.

RADIATION AND IMMUNOTHERAPY IN LOCALLY ADVANCED NON–SMALL CELL LUNG CANCER

Although there has been considerable interest in combining immunotherapy with RT in locally advanced NSCLC for the past several years,[44,45] the landmark PACIFIC trial made major strides in extending the use of checkpoint blockade strategies to earlier stage disease.[46] This double-blind, randomized phase 3 trial demonstrated improved OS as well as PFS in patients with locally advanced NSCLC treated with concurrent chemoradiation followed by the anti-PD-L1 antibody durvalumab. Two-year OS increased from 55% with standard therapy to 66% with durvalumab.[10] The 18-month PFS was similarly improved with addition of durvalumab (44.2% vs 27%). Interestingly, a subgroup analysis demonstrated that patients who were able to start adjuvant durvalumab within 14 days of completion of chemoradiation had improved OS and PFS compared with those who started after 14 days. Although these findings may only reflect that healthier patients were able

Table 1
Key recruiting or activating trials of combining radiation therapy and immunotherapy for metastatic non–small cell lung cancer

NCT Number/ Trial Name	Study Phase	N	Key Inclusion Criteria	IO Agent	Trial Design	RT Dose	RT and IO Timing	Status	Anticipated 1° Completion Date
Radiation to fewer than all sites of metastatic disease									
NCT02492568 PEMBRO-RT	2 Randomized	74	Stage IV NSCLC with minimum of 2 lesions; prior treatment with at least 1 line of chemotherapy	Pembrolizumab	IO ± SBRT up to 24 mo	SBRT 24 Gy/3 fx	RT completed first, with IO given within 7 d of the last fraction	Active, not recruiting	Jun 2018
NCT02658097 CASE1516	2 Randomized	48	Metastatic NSCLC with a minimum of 2 lesions	Pembrolizumab	IO ± SFRT (single-fraction RT)	8 Gy/1 fx	Concurrent (IO and RT to start on same day)	Recruiting	Dec 2019
NCT03044626 FORCE	2 Multicohort nonrandomized	130	Metastatic nonsquamous NSCLC with minimum of 2 lesions	Nivolumab	IO + concurrent RT (for patients who need RT) or IO monotherapy	20 Gy/5 fx to 1 metastasis	RT starts within 3 d of first IO dose	Recruiting	Aug 2019
NCT03176173 RRADICAL	2 Multicohort nonrandomized	85	Metastatic NSCLC with at least 1 extracranial lesion	Either nivolumab, pembrolizumab, or atezolizumab	IO ± SBRT	SBRT in up to 10 fractions	RT to start after a minimum of 4 wk IO	Recruiting	Jun 2020

(*continued on next page*)

Table 1
(continued)

NCT Number/ Trial Name	Study Phase	N	Key Inclusion Criteria	IO Agent	Trial Design	RT Dose	RT and IO Timing	Status	Anticipated 1° Completion Date
NCT02444741	1/2 Rando-mized	104	Stage IV NSCLC for phase 2 portion of trial with minimum of 2 lesions	Pembrolizumab	Multiple experimental groups with IO + either SBRT or wide field RT (WFRT)	SBRT to 50 Gy/4 fx, WFRT to 45 Gy/15 fx	Variable; some cohorts concurrent, some sequential with IO first, some with RT only after progression on IO	Recruiting	Sep 2020
NCT02239900	1/2 Randomized	120	Multiple solid tumor types, including NSCLC with at least 1 metastasis or 1° in lung, liver, or adrenal	Ipilimumab	Multiple experimental groups with IO + SBRT	SBRT to 50 Gy/4 fx or 60 Gy/10 fx. 1–4 lesions can be treated	Concurrent or with IO given for 2 cycles before SBRT	Active, not recruiting	Aug 2019
NCT03168464	1/2 Single arm	45	Metastatic NSCLC with a minimum of 2 lesions	Ipilimumab + nivolumab	IO + RT	30 Gy/5 fx to 1 lesions	Ipilimumab and RT start on same day, nivolumab added on day 22	Recruiting	Dec 2021
NCT03223155	1 Randomized	80	Stage IV NSCLC with a minimum of 2 lesions	Ipilimumab + nivolumab	SBRT + IO	SBRT in 3–5 fractions to 2–4 sites	Either concurrent IO + RT or sequential (IO to start 1–7 d after RT completed)	Recruiting	Dec 2020

NCT02400814	1 Multicohort nonrandomized	45	Stage IV or recurrent NSCLC with minimum of 2 lesions	Atezolizumab	IO + SBRT	SBRT in 5 fractions	3 cohorts, with concurrent, induction, and sequential timing of RT and IO	Active, not recruiting	Apr 2020
NCT03307759 SABRseq	1	32	Stage IV PD-L1$^+$ NSCLC with minimum of 2 lesions	Pembrolizumab	IO + SBRT	SBRT	Either SBRT followed by IO or IO followed by SBRT after cycle 1	Recruiting	Nov 2021
NCT03368222 PRIMING	1	24	Stage IV NSCLC or IIIB unable to be treated curatively	Pembrolizumab	IO + SBRT	SBRT to 30 Gy/3 fx or 54 Gy/3 fx or maximum tolerated dose	RT to start 14 d after IO	Active, not recruiting	Mar 2021
NCT03158883	1	26	Stage IV NSCLC with primary resistance or secondary progression on anti–PD-1 therapy	Avelumab	IO + SBRT	50 Gy/5 fx	Patients on IO for variable lengths of time before RT	Recruiting	Jun 2020
NCT03035890	N/A	33	Metastatic NSCLC with a minimum of 3 lesions	Either nivolumab, pembrolizumab, or atezolizumab	IO + SBRT	SBRT to either 24–45 Gy/3 fx, or 30–50 Gy/5 fx	Concurrent	Active, not recruiting	Dec 2019

(*continued on next page*)

Table 1
(continued)

NCT Number/ Trial Name	Study Phase	N	Key Inclusion Criteria	IO Agent	Trial Design	RT Dose	RT and IO Timing	Status	Anticipated 1° Completion Date
Radiation to all sites of oligometastatic disease									
NCT02316002	2 Single arm	51	Stage IV oligometastatic NSCLC with up to 4 mets; prior treatment with at least 1 line of chemotherapy	Pembrolizumab	IO + locally ablative therapy (LAT) to all sites of disease	RT, ablation, or surgery all allowed	LAT completed first, with IO given 4–12 wk after	Completed	Sep 2018
NCT03965468 CHESS	2	47	Stage IV oligometastatic NSCLC with up to 3 mets (one must be extracranial)	Durvalumab	IO + traditional chemotherapy, then RT to all mets. If no progression at 3 mo, RT or surgery to primary lung tumor	SBRT to a maximum of 10 fractions	RT to start after 1 wk of IO + traditional chemotherapy	Recruiting	Dec 2021
NCT03275597	1	21	Stage IV NSCLC with up to 6 extracranial mets	Durvalumab + tremelimumab	RT to all sites of disease followed by IO	SBRT to 30–50 Gy in 5 fractions	IO starts 7 d after RT	Recruiting	Oct 2020
NCT03867175	3	116	Stage IV oligometastatic NSCLC with up to 8 mets	Pembrolizumab	IO up to 1 year ± SBRT to all mets	SBRT in 3–10 fractions	Concurrent	Recruiting	Jul 2027

Abbreviations: fx, fractions; IO, immunotherapy; mets, metastases; N/A, not available.

to proceed to consolidative ICB therapy faster, they may also suggest an importance of initiating immunotherapy soon after RT for maximum benefit.

Further support of the benefit of combining immunotherapy with definitive treatment of locally advanced NSCLC comes from the Hoosier Cancer Network trial LUN14-179.[47] This phase 2 single-arm trial administered consolidative pembrolizumab to 93 patients who had not progressed 4 to 8 weeks after completion of concurrent chemoradiation. Interim results with a median follow-up of 16.4 months were reported at American Society of Clinical Oncology 2018. The 18-month PFS was 49.5%, and the estimated 2-year OS was 68.7%, similar to the outcomes reported on the PACIFIC trial with durvalumab and significantly better than historical controls. The median time to metastatic disease or death was not yet reached.

In the wake of the PACIFIC trial's success with consolidative therapy, clinicians are now exploring whether it is safe to use immunotherapy concurrently with chemoradiation (**Table 2**). It is possible that combined checkpoint blockade with chemotherapy and RT could lead to increased rates of pneumonitis, a serious complication in a patient population that often has impaired lung function at baseline. The PACIFIC trial excluded any patients with unresolved grade 2 toxicities caused by chemoradiation. With this design, overall rates of grade 3 or higher pneumonitis were low and similar between the durvalumab arm and the placebo arm (3.4% vs 2.1%, respectively).[10] The ETOP NICOLAS trial recently reported an interim safety analysis of moving immunotherapy to the upfront concurrent setting.[48] This single-arm phase 2 trial administered nivolumab at the same time as definitive chemoradiation to patients with locally advanced, unresectable NSCLC. At 3 months post-RT, none of the initial 21 patients experienced grade 3 or worse pneumonitis. Given this encouraging initial safety profile, a total of 80 patients were enrolled. Of these, 8 have experienced grade 3 or higher pneumonitis. This larger cohort will be evaluated for 1-year PFS.

A handful of trials will explore whether standard platinum-doublet chemotherapy can be replaced by immunotherapy in locally advanced NSCLC. The currently enrolling NRG Oncology LU004 ARCHON-1 trial will accrue 24 patients with high (>50%) PD-L1 staining on tumors and treat them with definitive thoracic radiation with concurrent durvalumab. Two radiation regimens will be trials: 60 Gy either in a conventional 30 fractions or hypofractionated RT in 15 fractions. This trial design builds upon results from the KEYNOTE-024 study, which saw improved OS and PFS with pembrolizumab versus standard chemotherapy as first-line therapy in patients with metastatic NSCLC and greater than 50% PD-L1 staining.[49]

The DART trial also omits chemotherapy from treatment of locally advanced NSCLC, but addresses a different patient subset. Because of medical comorbidities, up to 50% to 60% of patients with unresectable NSCLC are ineligible for standard concurrent chemoradiation. Although sequential use of chemotherapy followed by radiation is a less toxic (although less effective) alternative,[19] many patients unfit for the concurrent regimen receive RT alone with very limited chance of cure. Designed for this frailer cohort, the DART trial is a single-arm study with planned enrollment of 53 patients in which concurrent durvalumab and thoracic radiation to 60 Gy in 30 fractions will be administered, followed by a year of consolidative durvalumab.

Trials testing neoadjuvant strategies in resectable locally advanced NSCLC are also eagerly anticipated, not only for their possible efficacy data but also for the additional tissue obtained at surgery that can be used for correlative studies. In the phase 1 CASE 4516 trial (NCT02987998), 20 patients with stage 3A NSCLC will receive neoadjuvant chemoradiation with cisplatin, etoposide, and 45 Gy in 25 fractions along with pembrolizumab. They will then proceed to surgery followed by consolidation pembrolizumab. A phase 2 study (NCT03237377) will look at the effects of neoadjuvant durvalumab and radiation (45 Gy in 25 fractions) with neoadjuvant tremelimumab (a CTLA-4 inhibitor) added to an expansion cohort if the initial immunotherapy and RT combination appears safe. Patients will receive standard adjuvant chemotherapy if indicated. These studies will obtain tumor samples before and after treatment with RT and ICB, which may offer mechanistic insight into the interaction of the two therapies.

RADIATION AND IMMUNOTHERAPY IN EARLY-STAGE NON–SMALL CELL LUNG CANCER

There is currently little published experience on the combined use of RT and ICB in early-stage NSCLC. The focal therapies of surgical lobectomy and SBRT are the core treatments for this stage of disease, with local control rates of exceeding 90%. Traditional chemotherapeutic agents have historically played a limited role in early-stage disease. In fact, among stage I-III NSCLC patients undergoing surgical resection, a large metaanalysis demonstrated no OS benefit with the addition of

Table 2
Key recruiting or activating trials of combining radiation therapy and immunotherapy for locally advanced non–small cell lung cancer

NCT Number/ Trial Name	Study Phase	N	Key Inclusion Criteria	IO Agent	Trial Design	RT Dose	RT and IO Timing	Status	Anticipated 1° Completion Date
Definitive radiation									
NCT03519971 PACIFIC 2	3	328	Unresectable stage III NSCLC	Durvalumab	Concurrent IO + platinum-based chemoRT, followed by adjuvant IO	60 Gy/30 fx	Concurrent	Active, not recruiting	Aug 2022
NCT03693300 PACIFIC 6	2 Single arm	150	Unresectable stage III NSCLC in patients suitable for sequential platinum-based chemo-therapy + RT	Durvalumab	Sequential chemotherapy and thoracic radiation, followed by IO	60 Gy/30 fx	IO to start within 28 d after RT completion	Recruiting	Feb 2023
NCT02343952 HCRN LUN14–179	2 Single arm	93	Inoperable or unresectable stage IIIA/B NSCLC who have not progressed after chemoRT	Pembrolizumab	Platinum-based chemoRT, followed by consolidation IO up to 12 mo	Conventional RT to 59.4–66.6 Gy	IO to begin 28–56 d after chemoRT	Active, not recruiting (enrollment complete)	Sep 2020
NCT02434081 NICOLAS	2 Single arm	78	Unresectable stage IIIA/B NSCLC	Nivolumab	Standard chemoRT + IO concurrently and adjuvantly up to 12 mo	60 Gy/30 fx	Concurrent	Ongoing not recruiting	Aug 2020

NCT03102242	2 Single arm	63	Unresectable stage IIIA/B NSCLC	Atezolizumab	Induction IO for 4 cycles followed by carboplatin-based chemoRT, followed by adjuvant IO	60 Gy/30 fx	RT to start after 4 cycles IO	Recruiting	Mar 2020
NCT02525757 DETERRED	2 Multicohort nonrandomized	40	Unresectable stage II–III NSCLC	Atezolizumab	Carboplatin-based chemoRT ± IO, followed by 3–4 wk chemotherapy holiday (±1 dose IO), followed by 2 cycles consolidation traditional chemo + IO, followed by maintenance IO up to 12 mo	Conventional RT to 60–66 Gy	Concurrent therapy or RT completed first, depending on cohort	Active, not recruiting (enrollment complete)	Jan 2020
NCT03999710 DART	1/2 Single arm	53	Patients with unresectable stage III NSCLC not suitable for concurrent chemoradiation	Durvalumab	IO + RT (no traditional chemotherapy)	60 Gy/30 fx	RT started within 1 wk of durvalumab (preferably same day)	Recruiting	Jul 2021
NCT03801902 ARCHON-1	1 Single arm	24	Unresectable stage II–III NSCLC with high PD-L1 (>50%)	Durvalumab	IO + RT (no traditional chemotherapy)	Conventional RT to 60 Gy/30 fx or hypofractionated RT to 60 Gy/15 fx	RT to start 2 wk after first IO dose	Recruiting	Jul 2020

(*continued on next page*)

Table 2
(*continued*)

NCT Number/ Trial Name	Study Phase	N	Key Inclusion Criteria	IO Agent	Trial Design	RT Dose	RT and IO Timing	Status	Anticipated 1° Completion Date
NCT02621398	1 Multicohort nonrandomized	30	Unresectable stage II–III NSCLC	Pembrolizumab	Platinum-based chemoRT + IO	60 Gy/30 fx	IO (either full dose or reduced dose), started concurrently, at the penultimate week of RT, or 2–6 wk after RT completion depending on cohort	Active, not recruiting (enrollment complete)	Dec 2021
Neoadjuvant radiation									
NCT03237377	2 Single arm	32	Resectable stage IIIA NSCLC	Durvalumab ± tremelimumab	Neoadjuvant IO + RT, followed by surgery	45 Gy/25 fx	Concurrent	Recruiting	Sep 2021
NCT03053856	2 Single arm	37	Stage IIIA NSCLC with N2 disease	Pembrolizumab	Neoadjuvant chemoRT, followed by surgery, followed by adjuvant IO	44 Gy/22 fx	RT completed before surgery, IO given in adjuvant setting	Not yet recruiting	May 2021
NCT02987998 CASE4516	1	20	Resectable stage IIIA NSCLC	Pembrolizumab	Neoadjuvant chemoRT + IO, followed by surgery, followed by	45 Gy/25 fx	Concurrent	Recruiting	Jan 2024

					consolidation IO				
Adjuvant radiation									
NCT02572843	2 Single arm	68	Resectable stage IIIA NSCLC with N2 disease	Durvalumab	Neoadjuvant chemoRT, followed by neoadjuvant IO, then surgery. Postoperative R0 patients will receive adjuvant IO whereas R1/2 patients will receive RT followed by adjuvant IO	Conventional postoperative RT	IO begun before surgery; RT may be given postoperatively before additional adjuvant IO	Active, not recruiting	Mar 2021
Reirradiation for local recurrence									
NCT03087760	2 Single arm	41	Patients with prior chemoRT treatment of locally advanced NSCLC, now with local recurrence in/near prior RT field	Pembrolizumab	Concurrent chemo + proton RT, followed by up to 24 mo IO	Conventionally fractionated proton RT	RT completed first	Recruiting	Dec 2020

Table 3
Key recruiting or activating trials of combining radiation therapy and immunotherapy for early-stage non–small cell lung cancer

NCT Number/ Trial Name	Study Phase	N	Key Inclusion Criteria	IO Agent	Trial Design	RT Dose	RT and IO Timing	Status	Anticipated 1° Completion Date
Definitive radiation									
NCT03833154 PACIFIC 4	3	630	Stage I–II	Durvalumab	SBRT ± IO up to 24 mo	SBRT	RT completed first	Recruiting	Oct 2023
NCT03446547 ASTEROID	2 Randomized	216	Inoperable stage I NSCLC	Durvalumab	SBRT ± IO up to 12 mo	3 or 4 fractions RT	RT completed first	Recruiting	Dec 2021
NCT03110978 I-SABR	2 Randomized	140	Inoperable stage I and IIA NSCLC	Nivolumab	SBRT ± IO up to 3 mo	SBRT to 50 Gy/4 fx, or (if constraints cannot be met) 70 Gy/10 fx	Concurrent; IO to start within 36 h before or after the first SBRT fraction	Recruiting	Jun 2022
NCT03148327	1/2 Randomized	105	Inoperable stage I/IIA NSCLC	Durvalumab	SBRT ± IO up to 5 mo	SBRT to 54 Gy/3 fx, 50 Gy/4 fx, or 65 Gy/10 fx	IO starts first, RT to start between 5 and 10 d of first dose	Recruiting	Jun 2020
NCT03050554	1/2 Single arm	56	Inoperable stage I NSCLC	Avelumab	SBRT + IO up to 2 mo	SBRT to 50 Gy/5 fx or 48 Gy/4 fx	Concurrent	Active, not recruiting	Oct 2020
NCT03383302 STILE	1/2 Single arm	31	Inoperable stage I NSCLC	Nivolumab	SBRT + IO	SBRT in 3 or 5 fractions	RT completed first; IO to start within 24 h of last fraction	Recruiting	Jun 2021

NCT02599454	1	33	Inoperable stage I NSCLC	Atezolizumab	SBRT + IO	SBRT to 50 Gy in 4 or 5 fractions	3 cycles of IO, then RT to start within 24–48 h of third dose	Active, not recruiting	Sep 2020
Neoadjuvant radiation									
NCT02904954	2 Randomized	60	Resectable stage I–IIIA NSCLC	Durvalumab	Neoadjuvant IO ± SBRT, followed by surgery, followed by postoperative maintenance IO	SBRT to 24 Gy/3 fx	Concurrent	Recruiting	Jan 2020
NCT03217071 PembroX	2 Randomized	40	Resectable stage I–IIIA NSCLC	Pembrolizumab	Neoadjuvant IO ± SBRT, followed by surgery within 6 wk	SBRT to 12 Gy/1 fx delivered to 50% of the primary lung tumor	2 cycles of IO, then RT to start within 1 wk (±3 d) of second dose	Recruiting	Sep 2019
Adjuvant radiation									
NCT02818920 TOP 1501	2	32	Resectable stage I–IIIA NSCLC	Pembrolizumab	Neoadjuvant IO, followed by surgery, followed by adjuvant IO. Traditional adjuvant postoperative chemotherapy ± RT will also be given based on clinical scenario	Conventional postoperative RT	IO begun before surgery; RT may be given in adjuvant setting	Active, not recruiting	Mar 2019

chemotherapy in node-negative patients, but there was a significant benefit for node-positive, more advanced stage patients.[50] Randomized studies, however, have demonstrated a survival benefit to adjuvant chemotherapy following surgery for node-negative patients with tumors 4 cm or more.[51]

Similarly, although it is thought that adding cytotoxic chemotherapy to SBRT for small stage I NSCLC lesions increases toxicity without appreciable benefit, for large node-negative patients who are increasingly being treated with SBRT,[52,53] the addition of chemotherapy may improve OS.[54] For both surgical and SBRT patients with smaller node-negative tumors, they are still at relatively high risk for regional and distant recurrences, with 2-year PFS rates ranging from 60% to 80% in various studies.[55,56] Current National Comprehensive Cancer Network guidelines recommend observation for stage IA, IB, and IIA patients (American Joint Committee on Cancer, 8th Edition) following definitive local therapy, with consideration of adjuvant chemotherapy in select patients with certain high-risk features such as poorly differentiated tumors, tumors greater than 4 cm, positive lymphovascular invasion, wedge resection performed (vs the more definitive lobectomy), visceral pleural involvement, and unknown lymph node status. The potential benefits of adjuvant chemotherapy must be weighed even more carefully in medically inoperable early-stage patients who receive SBRT, because this frailer cohort may be more likely to experience adverse and potentially fatal toxicities from chemotherapy.

Given the clear threat of early dissemination of micrometastatic disease in NSCLC, several trials are now examining whether the addition of adjuvant immunotherapy following SBRT may improve PFS (**Table 3**). At least 7 trials are currently open that address this question, the largest of which is the phase 3 PACIFIC-4 trial that will randomize 630 patients to receive SBRT with or without adjuvant durvalumab for a total of 2 years. The related trial I-SABR requires nivolumab to be started concurrently with the first fraction of SBRT, which the trial defines as 36 hours before or after radiation initiation. The eligibility criteria for both PACIFIC-4 and I-SABR include all patients with tumors $\leq$7 cm and negative nodes.

The SWOG/NRG Oncology intergroup S1914 phase 3 480-patient trial, which randomizes patients to SBRT alone or induction atezolizumab and then SBRT during cycle 3 of immunotherapy, exploits the potential immunologic benefits of ICB before SBRT and allows for optimal patient convenience with only 8 total cycles of atezolizumab. This trial requires tumors to be $\geq$2 cm, possess a maximum standardized uptake value of $\geq$6.2, or histology to be moderately to poorly differentiated. These selection criteria should help identify those who would most benefit from the addition of a systemic agent to SBRT.

Two other interesting trials in early-stage NSCLC will incorporate neoadjuvant immunotherapy and SBRT. Investigators from Weill Medical College of Cornell University are recruiting to a planned 60-patient study of resectable stage I–IIIA NSCLC in which patients are randomized to receive neoadjuvant durvalumab followed by surgery or neoadjuvant durvalumab and SBRT during the first cycle of immunotherapy followed by lobectomy (NCT02904954). The PEMBRO-X trial will administer neoadjuvant pembrolizumab for 2 cycles, followed by randomization of patients to receive 12 Gy in a single fraction delivered to the lateral half of the tumor, then followed by lobectomy. These unique study designs will permit pathologic comparison of the tumors and their immune infiltrates after exposure to immunotherapy with or without RT.

FUTURE DIRECTION AND SUMMARY

The combination of RT and ICB shows promise across the full spectrum of NSCLC, from stage I to stage IV disease. Numerous questions remain regarding the optimal timing and sequencing and the optimal radiation dose and fractionation needed to prime the immune response to be optimally unleashed through checkpoint inhibitors. Future studies are also needed to assess if advanced radiation modalities like proton therapy allow for improved clinical synergy with immunotherapy. Clinicians eagerly await the results from the trials detailed above.

DISCLOSURE

The authors have nothing to disclose.

REFERENCES

1. Siegel RL, Miller KD, Jemal A. Cancer statistics, 2019. CA Cancer J Clin 2019;69(1):7–34.
2. National Comprehensive Cancer Network. Clinical practice guidelines in oncology: non-small cell lung cancer. Version 1.2020-November 6, 2019. Available at: https://www.nccn.org/professionals/physician_gls/pdf/nscl.pdf. Accessed November 19, 2019.
3. Schonewolf CA, Verma V, Post CM, et al. Outcomes of invasive mediastinal nodal staging versus positron emission tomography staging alone for early-stage non-small cell lung cancer treated with

stereotactic body radiation therapy. Lung Cancer 2018;117:53–9.
4. Ribas A, Wolchok JD. Cancer immunotherapy using checkpoint blockade. Science 2018;359(6382): 1350–5.
5. Herbst RS, Baas P, Kim D-W, et al. Pembrolizumab versus docetaxel for previously treated, PD-L1-positive, advanced non-small-cell lung cancer (KEYNOTE-010): a randomised controlled trial. Lancet 2016;387(10027):1540–50.
6. Brahmer J, Reckamp KL, Baas P, et al. Nivolumab versus docetaxel in advanced squamous-cell non–small-cell lung cancer. N Engl J Med 2015;373(2): 123–35.
7. Borghaei H, Paz-Ares L, Horn L, et al. Nivolumab versus docetaxel in advanced nonsquamous non-small-cell lung cancer. N Engl J Med 2015;373(17): 1627–39.
8. Rittmeyer A, Barlesi F, Waterkamp D, et al. Atezolizumab versus docetaxel in patients with previously treated non-small-cell lung cancer (OAK): a phase 3, open-label, multicentre randomised controlled trial. Lancet 2017;389(10066):255–65.
9. Reck M, Rodríguez-Abreu D, Robinson AG, et al. Pembrolizumab versus chemotherapy for PD-L1-positive non-small-cell lung cancer. N Engl J Med 2016;375(19):1823–33.
10. Antonia SJ, Villegas A, Daniel D, et al. Overall survival with durvalumab after chemoradiotherapy in stage III NSCLC. N Engl J Med 2018;379(24): 2342–50.
11. Chang JY, Senan S, Paul MA, et al. Stereotactic ablative radiotherapy versus lobectomy for operable stage I non-small-cell lung cancer: a pooled analysis of two randomised trials. Lancet Oncol 2015;16(6): 630–7.
12. Choi JI, Simone CB 2nd. Stereotactic body radiation therapy versus surgery for early stage non-small cell lung cancer: clearing a path through an evolving treatment landscape. J Thorac Dis 2019;11(Suppl 9):S1360–5.
13. Simone CB 2nd, Dorsey JF. Additional data in the debate on stage I non-small cell lung cancer: surgery versus stereotactic ablative radiotherapy. Ann Transl Med 2015;3(13):172.
14. Videtic GMM, Donington J, Giuliani M, et al. Stereotactic body radiation therapy for early-stage non-small cell lung cancer: executive summary of an ASTRO evidence-based guideline. Pract Radiat Oncol 2017;7(5):295–301.
15. Albain KS, Swann RS, Rusch VW, et al. Radiotherapy plus chemotherapy with or without surgical resection for stage III non-small-cell lung cancer: a phase III randomised controlled trial. Lancet 2009; 374(9687):379–86.
16. Vyfhuis MAL, Burrows WM, Bhooshan N, et al. Implications of pathological complete response (pCR) beyond mediastinal nodal clearance with high-dose neoadjuvant chemoradiotherapy (CRT) in locally advanced, non-small cell lung cancer (LA-NSCLC). Int J Radiat Oncol Biol Phys 2018;101(2): 445–52.
17. Robinson CG, Patel AP, Bradley JD, et al. Postoperative radiotherapy for pathologic N2 non-small-cell lung cancer treated with adjuvant chemotherapy: a review of the National Cancer Data Base. J Clin Oncol 2015;33(8):870–6.
18. Bradley JD, Paulus R, Komaki R, et al. Standard-dose versus high-dose conformal radiotherapy with concurrent and consolidation carboplatin plus paclitaxel with or without cetuximab for patients with stage IIIA or IIIB non-small-cell lung cancer (RTOG 0617): a randomised, two-by-two factorial phase 3 study. Lancet Oncol 2015;16(2):187–99.
19. Aupérin A, Péchoux CL, Rolland E, et al. Meta-analysis of concomitant versus sequential radiochemotherapy in locally advanced non-small-cell lung cancer. J Clin Oncol 2010;28(13):2181–90.
20. Simone CB 2nd, Jones JA. Palliative care for patients with locally advanced and metastatic non-small cell lung cancer. Ann Palliat Med 2013;2(4): 178–88.
21. Jones JA, Simone CB 2nd. Palliative radiotherapy for advanced malignancies in a changing oncologic landscape: guiding principles and practice implementation. Ann Palliat Med 2014;3(3): 192–202.
22. Gomez DR, Tang C, Zhang J, et al. Local consolidative therapy vs. maintenance therapy or observation for patients with oligometastatic non-small-cell lung cancer: long-term results of a multi-institutional, phase II, randomized study. J Clin Oncol 2019; 37(18):1558–65.
23. Palma DA, Olson R, Harrow S, et al. Stereotactic ablative radiotherapy versus standard of care palliative treatment in patients with oligometastatic cancers (SABR-COMET): a randomised, phase 2, open-label trial. Lancet 2019; 393(10185):2051–8.
24. Sharma P, Hu-Lieskovan S, Wargo JA, et al. Primary, adaptive, and acquired resistance to cancer immunotherapy. Cell 2017;168(4):707–23.
25. Grassberger C, Ellsworth SG, Wilks MQ, et al. Assessing the interactions between radiotherapy and antitumour immunity. Nat Rev Clin Oncol 2019; 16(12):729–45.
26. Postow MA, Callahan MK, Barker CA, et al. Immunologic correlates of the abscopal effect in a patient with melanoma. N Engl J Med 2012;366(10): 925–31.
27. Barsky AR, Cengel KA, Katz SI, et al. First-ever abscopal effect after palliative radiotherapy and immuno-gene therapy for malignant pleural mesothelioma. Cureus 2019;11(2):e4102.

28. Bitran J. The abscopal effect exists in non-small cell lung cancer: a case report and review of the literature. Cureus 2019;11(2):e4118.
29. Twyman-Saint Victor C, Rech AJ, Maity A, et al. Radiation and dual checkpoint blockade activate non-redundant immune mechanisms in cancer. Nature 2015;520(7547):373–7.
30. Deng L, Liang H, Burnette B, et al. Irradiation and anti-PD-L1 treatment synergistically promote anti-tumor immunity in mice. J Clin Invest 2014;124(2):687–95.
31. Fujimoto D, Uehara K, Sato Y, et al. Alteration of PD-L1 expression and its prognostic impact after concurrent chemoradiation therapy in non-small cell lung cancer patients. Sci Rep 2017;7(1):11373.
32. Badiyan SN, Roach MC, Chuong MD, et al. Combining immunotherapy with radiation therapy in thoracic oncology. J Thorac Dis 2018;10(Suppl 21):S2492–507.
33. Simone CB 2nd, Berman AT, Jabbour SK. Harnessing the potential synergy of combining radiation therapy and immunotherapy for thoracic malignancies. Transl Lung Cancer Res 2017;6(2):109–12.
34. Simone CB 2nd, Burri SH, Heinzerling JH. Novel radiotherapy approaches for lung cancer: combining radiation therapy with targeted and immunotherapies. Transl Lung Cancer Res 2015;4(5):545–52.
35. Shaverdian N, Lisberg AE, Bornazyan K, et al. Previous radiotherapy and the clinical activity and toxicity of pembrolizumab in the treatment of non-small-cell lung cancer: a secondary analysis of the KEYNOTE-001 phase 1 trial. Lancet Oncol 2017;18(7):895–903.
36. Samstein R, Rimner A, Barker CA, et al. Combined immune checkpoint blockade and radiation therapy: timing and dose fractionation associated with greatest survival duration among over 750 treated patients. Int J Radiat Oncol Biol Phys 2017;99(2):S129–30.
37. Tang C, Welsh JW, de Groot P, et al. Ipilimumab with stereotactic ablative radiation therapy: phase I results and immunologic correlates from peripheral T cells. Clin Cancer Res 2017;23(6):1388–96.
38. Formenti SC, Rudqvist NP, Golden E, et al. Radiotherapy induces responses of lung cancer to CTLA-4 blockade. Nat Med 2018;24(12):1845–51.
39. Govindan R, Szczesna A, Ahn MJ, et al. Phase III trial of ipilimumab combined with paclitaxel and carboplatin in advanced squamous non-small-cell lung cancer. J Clin Oncol 2017;35(30):3449–57.
40. Theelen W, Peulen HMU, Lalezari F, et al. Effect of pembrolizumab after stereotactic body radiotherapy vs pembrolizumab alone on tumor response in patients with advanced non-small cell lung cancer: results of the PEMBRO-RT phase 2 randomized clinical trial. JAMA Oncol 2019. [Epub ahead of print].
41. Welsh JW, Menon H, Tang C, et al. Randomized phase I/II trial of pembrolizumab with and without radiotherapy for metastatic non-small cell lung cancer. J Clin Oncol 2019;37(15_suppl):9104.
42. Bauml JM, Mick R, Ciunci C, et al. Pembrolizumab after completion of locally ablative therapy for oligometastatic non-small cell lung cancer: a phase 2 trial. JAMA Oncol 2019. [Epub ahead of print].
43. Amin NP, Remick J, Agarwal M, et al. Concurrent radiation and immunotherapy: survey of practice patterns in the United States. Am J Clin Oncol 2019;42(2):208–14.
44. Berman AT, Simone CB 2nd. Immunotherapy in locally-advanced non-small cell lung cancer: releasing the brakes on consolidation? Transl Lung Cancer Res 2016;5(1):138–42.
45. Jabbour SK, Berman AT, Simone CB 2nd. Integrating immunotherapy into chemoradiation regimens for medically inoperable locally advanced non-small cell lung cancer. Transl Lung Cancer Res 2017;6(2):113–8.
46. Antonia SJ, Villegas A, Daniel D, et al. Durvalumab after chemoradiotherapy in stage III non-small-cell lung cancer. N Engl J Med 2017;377(20):1919–29.
47. Durm GA, Althouse SK, Sadiq AA, et al. Phase II trial of concurrent chemoradiation with consolidation pembrolizumab in patients with unresectable stage III non-small cell lung cancer: Hoosier Cancer Research Network LUN 14-179. J Clin Oncol 2018;36(15_suppl):8500.
48. Peters S, Felip E, Dafni U, et al. Safety evaluation of nivolumab added concurrently to radiotherapy in a standard first line chemo-radiotherapy regimen in stage III non-small cell lung cancer-The ETOP NICOLAS trial. Lung Cancer 2019;133:83–7.
49. Gottfried M. OA 17.06 - Updated Analysis of KEYNOTE-024: Pembrolizumab vs Platinum-Based Chemotherapy for Advanced NSCLC With PD-L1 TPS ≥50%. Paper presented at: 18th World Conference on Lung Cancer. Yokohama, Japan, October 18, 2017.
50. Pignon JP, Tribodet H, Scagliotti GV, et al. Lung adjuvant cisplatin evaluation: a pooled analysis by the LACE Collaborative Group. J Clin Oncol 2008;26(21):3552–9.
51. Strauss GM, Herndon JE 2nd, Maddaus MA, et al. Adjuvant paclitaxel plus carboplatin compared with observation in stage IB non-small-cell lung cancer: CALGB 9633 with the Cancer and Leukemia Group B, Radiation Therapy Oncology Group, and North Central Cancer Treatment Group Study Groups. J Clin Oncol 2008;26(31):5043–51.
52. Verma V, Shostrom VK, Kumar SS, et al. Multi-institutional experience of stereotactic body radiotherapy

for large (≥5 centimeters) non-small cell lung tumors. Cancer 2017;123(4):688–96.
53. Verma V, Shostrom VK, Zhen W, et al. Influence of fractionation scheme and tumor location on toxicities after stereotactic body radiation therapy for large (≥5 cm) non-small cell lung cancer: a multi-institutional analysis. Int J Radiat Oncol Biol Phys 2017;97(4):778–85.
54. Verma V, McMillian MT, Grover S, et al. Stereotactic body radiation therapy and the influence of chemotherapy on overall survival for large (≥5 centimeter) non-small cell lung cancer. Int J Radiat Oncol Biol Phys 2017;97(1):146–54.
55. Nakamura M, Nishikawa R, Mayahara H, et al. Pattern of recurrence after CyberKnife stereotactic body radiotherapy for peripheral early non-small cell lung cancer. J Thorac Dis 2019;11(1):214–21.
56. Senthi S, Lagerwaard FJ, Haasbeek CJ, et al. Patterns of disease recurrence after stereotactic ablative radiotherapy for early stage non-small-cell lung cancer: a retrospective analysis. Lancet Oncol 2012;13(8):802–9.

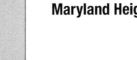

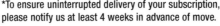

Printed and bound by CPI Group (UK) Ltd, Croydon, CR0 4YY

08/05/2025

01864694-0012